T0156502

Beyond the Knife

Alternatives to Surgery

Alan M. Lazar, MD, FACS
with Maury M. Breecher, PhD, MPH

Foreword by Stephen Sampson, DO

iUniverse, Inc.
Bloomington

Beyond the Knife
Alternatives to Surgery

iUniverse books may be ordered through booksellers or by contacting:

iUniverse
1663 Liberty Drive
Bloomington, IN 47403
www.iuniverse.com
1-800-Authors (1-800-288-4677)

ISBN: 978-1-4620-1767-6 (sc)
ISBN: 978-1-4620-1768-3 (dj)
ISBN: 978-1-4620-1769-0 (e)

Library of Congress Control Number: 2011906650

Printed in the United States of America

iUniverse rev. date: 7/26/2011

Dedication

I dedicate this book to several family members, both living and deceased; my brother Norman recently left us. I will always remember his love, friendship, advice, and his encouragement. Next, my wife, Barbara, whose love and partnership I cherish. I also dedicate this work to our children—Jaime, Jon, and Ali—who make my life complete. They should know how proud I am of them for their maturity, accomplishments, and compassion.

Alan M. Lazar, MD, FACS

I dedicate this book to my sons—Martin, Chris, and Michael—because I love them so much. I also dedicate this book to my grandchildren, Katelyn and Kevin. By the time you grow up, the future described in chapter 10 will have arrived.

Maury M. Breecher, PhD, MPH

Foreword

by Steve Sampson, DO

As fellow physicians specializing in musculoskeletal pain, Dr. Lazar and I mutually recognize that surgery may not always be the best alternative.

Dr. Lazar's book is the first to explain the tremendous medical advances make certain orthopedic surgeries obsolete. Within the last few years, exciting new treatments have been developed to eliminate the need for surgery in many conditions for which surgery was, in the past, the only option. Now, however, compelling research studies suggest the benefits of *Beyond the Knife* alternatives to surgery.

Dr. Lazar doesn't make any outlandish claims. He realizes surgery has its place in the practice of medicine but feels it is essential for patients to know when and if they have nonsurgical options. *Beyond the Knife* is well researched, evidenced by the many references cited.

When you read this book, you will learn about many cutting-edge therapies providing alternatives to surgery. Dr. Lazar has been an orthopedic surgeon for thirty years. He has always had a pioneering spirit while providing the very best of care to his patients even when the very best turns out not to include surgery. Patients have the right to be informed of their available treatment options, and in this book, Dr. Lazar allows them to make a knowledgeable choice about their health. Indeed, we have entered a new era—an era that goes *Beyond the Knife.*

Acknowledgements

A book of this scope cannot be created without the help of many learned people. My coauthor, science writer Maury Breecher, PhD, MPH, was invaluable in the brainstorming and creation process. Our medical library researcher, Vince Mariano, was persistent in our search for cutting-edge research articles. I thank our copy editor, Judith Lickus. I also thank Doctor Steve Sampson and Doctor David Crane for their knowledge and intellectual stimulation.

Table of Contents

Introduction

Introducing
Beyond the Knife Therapies

Being an orthopedic surgeon has placed me on the cutting edge (no pun intended) of medicine for over thirty years. As a surgeon, I realize that surgery is limited. I don't think most patients realize that surgery can leave them vulnerable to many serious infections, or that it neither guarantees nor even encourages healing. It's the natural healing mechanisms of the body that repair and mend any injury, pathology, or surgical trauma.

Consequently, one of the most important trends to emerge in medicine in recent years is that certain types of surgery are no longer necessary for many injuries, ailments, and conditions for which, in the recent past, surgery was the only option.

This is vital information for people considering surgery, yet it hasn't had wide publicity in newspapers, magazines, or on television or the Internet. It is truly a medical trend about which *many doctors, especially surgeons, don't want you to know.*

Depending on your doctor, you might not be told of this trend. So, join me as we go *Beyond the Knife* to explore some of the many possibilities instead of surgery that exist today thanks to inquisitive minds who knew there had to be a better way.

Treatments like platelet rich plasma (PRP) and adult stem-cell (ASC) therapies may be used to treat injuries to various body parts and also tighten and grow cartilage joints in shoulders, hips, and knees. More and more scientific studies suggest biologically based therapies, including PRP; heal injuries suffered by professional athletes, "weekend warriors," and even those suffering from arthritis. There is a growing need for new nonsurgical treatment options given the increasingly active baby boomer population and its overwhelming demand for total joint replacements.

You will learn about real people, some of the medical challenges they faced, and surgeries they avoided. Be prepared for the exciting adventure of discovering myriad therapies, treatments, and approaches that can be used to avoid surgery.

For instance, in my own practice, instead of surgery I often use platelet rich plasma (PRP) and adult stem cells (ASCs), which work together to heal arthritic joints, including osteoarthritis in the hip and knee; sports injuries, including tendonitis (tennis and golfer's elbow) and torn ligaments; back pain, hard-to-heal meniscal tears (tears in knee tissue and cartilage); rotator cuff injuries; and many more conditions involving the musculoskeletal system (bones, joints, muscles, ligaments, and tendons).

In chapters 2–5, you will learn how PRP and ASC therapies promote safe and effective natural healing for many of those conditions.

As a physician, my primary oath is, "First do no harm" so, whenever possible, we begin with the least invasive treatments. Those less-intrusive therapies may include acupuncture, energy healing, physical therapy, modification of activity levels, and exercises designed to build muscles around the injured part. We are now beginning to appreciate the value of less invasive complementary and nontraditional medical treatments as alternatives to surgery. In Chapter 6 you will read more about those exciting treatments.

Physicians are also beginning to understand the importance of nutritional supplementation in preventing surgery, especially for osteoarthritis-related ailments. Chapter 7 provides you with as much information on nutritional information as some other entire books do. That chapter discusses the use of natural anti-inflammatory agents, including vitamin/mineral supplementation ranging from glucosamine and chondroitin for joint protection to resveratrol for its beneficial anti-aging effects and cardio protection.

Other *Beyond the Knife* alternatives to surgery include better chemotherapies to prevent colorectal surgery, laser therapies to prevent diabetic amputations, and bio-identical estrogen and hormone replacement therapies to prevent osteoporosis-related surgeries.

Among the new *Beyond the Knife* therapies are *cryotherapy,* used to treat prostate, liver, and breast cancers; *extracorporeal shock wave therapy* for kidney stones and heel spurs; and *radiofrequency ablation* for varicose veins and supraventricular tachyarrhythmias. Chapter 8 provides a comprehensive roundup of those treatments.

We conclude our *Beyond the Knife* roundup with a look at some even more fantastic potential substitutes for surgery by exploring the promise of both genetic engineering and nanotechnology. Nanotechnology and gene therapy promise even more breakthroughs in the near future. Chapter 9 will be your "crystal ball" describing current and future breakthroughs in those fields.

Take-Home Points from the Introduction:

- Certain types of surgery are no longer necessary for many injuries, ailments, and conditions for which, in the recent past, surgery was the only option.

- Two *Beyond the Knife* therapies, platelet rich plasma (PRP) and adult stem cells (ASCs) work together to heal arthritic joints, including osteoarthritis in the hip and knee; sports injuries, including tendonitis (tennis and golfer's elbow) and torn ligaments; back pain; hard-to-heal meniscal tears (tears in knee tissue and cartilage); rotator cuff injuries; and many more conditions involving the musculoskeletal system (bones, joints, muscles, ligaments, tendons).

- Both PRP and ASCs encourage healing.

1

Why You Should Go
Beyond the Knife to Avoid Surgery

Have you seen the following headlines?

"Hospital-Acquired Superbug Infections Soar…"[1]
"Lax Infection Control at Surgery Centers" [2]
"Staph Infection Risk Rises with Brain, Chest Surgeries"[3]

Aren't those headlines scary? Their common message is that surgery is a leading cause of staph infections. They occur after many types of surgery especially brain and chest surgery, and after orthopaedic and plastic surgery.[4] Further evidence is highlighted by the Consumer's Union citing the U.S. Centers for Disease Control and Prevention (CDC)[5] which says that more than 290,000 surgical site infections occur in U.S. hospitals each year. Surgical wounds become infected with staph or other germs, killing thousands of people each year, according to the US Centers for Disease Control and Prevention (CDC).[6] Not surprising since the CDC also estimates that 25 percent to 30 percent of the American Population are carriers of staph infections.[7]

The first headline above reports that not even our newborn babies are safe because the MRSA "Super Bug" has increased "over 300 percent in U.S. newborn care units (NICUs) in the past ten years."[8] MRSA stands for methicillin-resistant staphylococcus aureus. This antibiotic resistant infection is notoriously hard to treat.

Studies have shown that MRSA exacts a heavy financial toll. Patients infected with MRSA after surgery spend an additional three weeks in the hospital and cost an additional $60,000 to care for.[9] Furthermore, compared with patients who go home from surgery uninfected, patients with MRSA infections are thirty-five times more likely to be readmitted to the hospital and seven times more likely to die within three months.[10]

According to one study, almost 32 percent of patients who developed MRSA pneumonia died in hospital during that admission. Vancomycin, the only drug effective against MRSA, is unlikely to boost survival since it is associated with more adverse effects such as renal toxicity but not with improved survival.[11]

Headlines such as those reveal a simple fact: surgery is dangerous. It sometimes even results in death. Surgeries can also cause pain, scarring, and disfiguration. For those reasons, surgery should never be decided on without knowledge of its risks and the effectiveness of any available *Beyond the Knife* alternatives.

Don't get me wrong. Surgery still has a vital role in medicine. There is no doubt that in cases of malignancy, such as cancerous tumors and in cases of severe physical trauma, surgery can be a lifesaver.

However, doctors are now realizing that surgical site infections (SSIs) are a real risk associated with any surgical procedure. They, "represent a significant burden in terms of patient morbidity (illness) and mortality (death), and cost to health services around the world."[12] An estimated 2.6 percent of nearly thirty million surgical operations get SSIs every year, according to the Institute for Healthcare Improvement. Each infection is estimated by the Institute to increase a hospital stay by an average of seven days and add over $3,000 in charges.[13]

SSIs refer to the sites of surgical incisions. The phrase, "surgical site infection," came into being in 1992, when the CDC revised its definition of "wound infection" and created the definition "surgical site infection" to prevent confusion between the infection of a surgical incision and the infection of a traumatic wound. Most SSIs are superficial, but even so, they contribute greatly to morbidity and mortality, according to three creators of a medical website dedicated to providing an overview of SSIs.[14]

Other Risks of Surgery

All surgeries have a risk of death, but some types have higher risks than others. For instance, during open-heart surgeries, the heart is actually stopped for almost an hour before being restarted. Obviously, that surgery has a higher risk than surgeries in which the heart is not stopped.

Furthermore, when undergoing any surgery, an individual faces the additional risk that internal organs may be damaged. For instance, a patient having an appendectomy (removal of their appendix) may incur an accidental injury to the intestine, which is attached to the appendix. That sort of injury is usually detected during the surgery and fixed immediately. However, if it is not, the intestine can become infected, and the infection can spread throughout the body. This can be life threatening.

Elderly people and those who are obese and/or have type II diabetes are at increased risk from surgery. Among those risks are SSIs, excessive bleeding, anesthesia complications, blood clots, and interior and exterior scarring.

— The Risks of Anesthesia during Surgery

Drugs used in general anesthesia are thought to cause injury to brain cells.[15] Consequently, medical experts have speculated that the dangers of the use of anesthetics include memory loss, an increased risk of Alzheimer's disease,[16] and, in children, may even interfere with brain development.

Anesthesia involves exposing your body to controlled levels of toxic chemicals in order to cause you to enter an unconscious state. One of the most common dangers of anesthesia is an allergic reaction to one of the chemicals used to induce this unconsciousness. All anesthetics, even a local one, can carry the risk of allergic reaction. In high doses, local anesthetics can cause toxic effects, since the chemicals are being absorbed through the skin and spread throughout the body by the bloodstream. Anesthesia, even local or regional anesthesia, can significantly affect your breathing, heartbeat, blood pressure, and other vital bodily functions.

— Intubation Difficulties that May Occur During Anesthesia

Many of the problems associated with anesthesia are often caused by the process of intubation, the insertion of the breathing tube. Breathing tubes are necessary because a person deprived of oxygen for four to six minutes can experience brain death. Longer periods without air lead to heart failure. To protect against that occurrence, the anesthesiologist inserts a breathing tube, called an endotracheal tube, into the windpipe. Just behind the windpipe's tracheal opening is the esophagus. If this tube is mistakenly inserted into the esophagus, oxygen will not be delivered to the lungs. After a few minutes, the patient will turn blue and suffer cardiac arrest, unless the condition is rapidly identified and rectified.

Some patients have throat and airway abnormalities that may make the placement of the airway tube hard or even impossible to accomplish. Repeated attempts to intubate the patient can lead to airway trauma that could interfere with the patient's ability to breathe. If that occurs, another surgical operation, an emergency tracheotomy (a hole in the windpipe), has to be accomplished quickly, or the patient will die.

Trained anesthesiologists have sophisticated equipment to prevent misplacement of the endotracheal tube. However, if that equipment is not present, say in a doctor's office where surgery is performed or if it is not working, or the airway tube is being inserted by someone not as well trained as an anesthesiologist, misplacement may occur and hypoxia (lack of oxygen) would result.

Other Problems Involving Anesthesia during Surgery

— *Aspiration*

Aspiration, the breathing of fluid into the lungs, can be a life-threatening problem when intubated. That's why patients are told not to eat or drink anything for several hours before surgery. Pregnant patients, very obese patients, trauma victims, and patients with bowel obstructions are the most at-risk groups for aspiration.

— *Nerve Damage*

Even local or regional anesthetics can, in rare cases, cause nerve damage, including persistent numbness, weakness, or pain. For most patients, those symptoms are temporary conditions, but some unlucky patients may experience these symptoms as permanent complications.

— *Ventilation Problems*

Once the airway tube is in place, oxygen and other gas exchanges need to occur so that oxygen is delivered to the body and carbon dioxide is removed.

This is usually accomplished by the use of a device known as a ventilator. Although it is a normal procedure for an anesthesiologist to introduce paralyzing drugs to the patient to keep him or her immobile, deeply anesthetized paralyzed patients are not able to breathe on their own. If the ventilator malfunctions or anything else interferes with this normal exchange of gases, the patient can rapidly be in severe danger from hypoxia.

Still More Life-Threatening Conditions Associated with Surgery

— *Blood Circulation Problems during Surgery*

Many anesthetic drugs can interfere with blood circulation. Anesthetics are all toxic in amounts slightly higher than those that produce unconsciousness, thus, their administration is a balancing act between unconsciousness and death. An overdose can stop the heart. However, a "normal" dose of various anesthetics can also lead to heart stoppage if the patient has a low threshold for that type of drug.

— *Blood Clots, Excessive Bleeding, and Infections from Transfusions after Major Surgery*

After major surgery, many postoperative patients are given medications to thin their blood and prevent the formation of clots. Clotting can become a critical complication if the clots travel through the bloodstream and lodge in the lung, a condition known as pulmonary embolism, or the brain, causing a stroke.

One type of blood clot is particularly dangerous. It is known as deep venous thrombosis (DVT). It can occur after any surgical operation, but is more likely to occur following surgery on the knee, hip, or pelvis. A DVT can cause the leg or legs to swell and become painful and warm to the touch. Like other clots, it could lodge in the lungs or brain.

— *Excessive Bleeding*

Another blood-related risk is excessive bleeding. This can be severe enough to necessitate a transfusion. Although the nation's blood supply is very safe, HIV, hepatitis A and B, and other viruses can be transferred during transfusions.

— *Paralysis Caused by Surgery*

Although rare, one of the most severe complications that can occur during surgery is permanent paralysis. However, it can occur, particularly during spinal or brain surgery.

– *Numbness, Tingling and Pain after Surgery*

Many surgical patients experience numbness, tingling, and pain after surgery. These sensations generally go away within a few days. However, a very small percentage of patients will experience those sensations for the rest of their lives!

– *Delayed Healing after Surgery*

Certain patients take longer to heal than others. People with co-morbidities (other illnesses, such as diabetes, hypertension, or an immune disorder) may have a longer, more painful recovery period. People with diabetes whose blood sugar levels are poorly controlled are likely to experience delayed healing after surgery. Consequently, people with diabetes must carefully consider the risks and rewards of any surgical procedure.

Conclusion

Surgery, when needed, can be life enhancing or even lifesaving. However, there are dangers to any surgery; no surgery is risk free. Surgery should be avoided when it can be. Alternatives to surgery, if available, should be considered. Those alternatives are the subject of the remainder of this book.

Take-Home Points from Chapter 1

- Surgery can leave one vulnerable to many serious infections and can neither guarantee nor even promote healing.
- Surgery should be avoided when it can be.
- Alternatives to surgery, when available, should be considered.

2

Introducing Stem-Cell Therapies and Platelet Rich Plasma

Do you recollect the toys called Transformers? They were neat because they could *transform* from toy cars, trucks, tanks, and other pieces of equipment into giant good guys—fighters against evil. Did you know that there are cells within the adult human body that have the same transformative powers?

Those cells are named stem cells. They are the pluripotent progenitors from which all other cells—blood cells, skeletal cells, vascular smooth muscle cells, muscle (skeletal and cardiac muscle), and adipocytes (fat tissue) cells—originate.

There are two types of stem cells: those that come from embryos and those that come from your own body. I do *not* use cells taken from embryos because of all the ethical, legal, religious, and political controversies that swirl around that type of stem cell. Instead, I use the second type, those known as adult stem cells (ASCs).

There are two types of ASCs:

1) *Hematopoietic cells,* from which all other blood-related cells are derived,[17] and

2) *Mesenchyme stem cells* (MSCs), which are undifferentiated cells from which all other cells are derived.

Hematopoietic cells have been used for many years in the treatment of a variety of malignant and nonmalignant blood-related conditions, solid tumors, and autoimmune diseases. The beneficial roles MSCs play have only recently been recognized.

The MSCs I use are harvested from the patient's own bone marrow or adipose tissues (fat cells).

ASCs from either source are little miracle workers because they are pluripotent. That means they have the capacity to give rise to the committed stem cells that make all other types of cells, platelets, or intermediary products during the body's own tissue repair process.

Our bodies are made up of billions and billions of cells, but by far, the vast majority of those cells are not stem cells because they have differentiated. That means that they have turned into specific types of cells. Skin cells, nerve cells, and heart cells are just three examples.

ASCs, however, are undifferentiated, which means they still have the ability to turn into any other type of cell. This has great ramifications for healing.

The Use of ASCs in Regenerative Medicine

ASCs are ideal candidates for use in regenerative medicine, tissue engineering, and bone cell replacement therapies because of their amazing ability to transform into various types of cells. The even have the ability to heal injured heart tissue,[18] thus potentially eliminating the need for certain types of cardiac surgery. This is huge. Heart disease remains the number one killer in the United States, according to the CDC. Every 25 seconds, an American will have a coronary event (a heart attack).[19]

"Numerous references now document the ability of these adult stem cells (ASCs) to contribute to the regeneration of cardiac tissue and improve performance of damaged hearts," according to Pessina and Grlbaldo, noted Italian researchers.[20] They add, "Results from clinical trials indicate that . . . [adult] stem cells … from the patients themselves, can regenerate damaged cardiac tissue and improve cardiac performance in humans."[21]

Here's a quote from a team of Hong Kong medical researchers about the importance of stem cells to cardiac therapy:

"Results of experimental studies have shown that after an intramyocardial (within the heart) infarction (this is doctor speak for a heart attack), implantation of bone marrow cells induces neovascularization (growth of new blood vessels), and improves heart function.[22]

Their study was of eight severe heart disease patients, all of whom were treated with injections of their own stem cells to eleven specific regions of the heart. After three months of follow-up, "There was improvement in symptoms, myocardial perfusion [blood flow in the heart], and function," wrote the researchers from Hong Kong.[23]

Both the Italian and the Hong Kong medical investigators are saying that bone marrow cells (ASCs) induced the growth of needed new blood vessels in the heart and improved heart function after a heart attack.

That's exciting stuff. Coronary artery disease remains a major cause of injury and death in the Western world. Any therapy that shows signs of combating coronary artery disease should be well studied and used when appropriate.

ASCs can save lives and improve quality of life (QoL) when used to treat many disorders. For instance, the authors of the earlier cited *Current Medical Research and Opinions* article also points out, "Genetically-engineered human adult stem cells have already been used in the successful treatment of patients with genetic disease. Bone marrow stem cells … were removed from the patients, a functional gene inserted, and the engineered cells reintroduced to the same patients. The stem cells … corrected the defect."[24]

That's more exciting information that backs up the usefulness of ASCs. There have also been reports of using ASCs to accelerate wound healing in patients with skin cancer and in those with chronic, nonhealing lower extremity wounds, such as diabetic leg ulcers.[25]

Platelet Rich Plasma and Stem-Cell Therapies

PRP and stem-cell therapy are often used together to achieve miraculous healings.

PRP and stem-cell treatments (utilizing stem cells from your own body) are among the most promising of the many *Beyond the Knife* therapies that encourage the body to heal itself without surgery.

– What Is Platelet Rich Plasma?

PRP is a concentrated blood sample of platelets from the patient's own blood. That concentrated clear plasma portion of the blood usually contains four to five times the amount of platelets normally found in blood.

Autologous (from your own blood) PRP is increasingly used in almost all fields of surgery for the clinical treatment of a variety of soft and hard tissue applications, most notably in accelerating bone formation and in the management of chronic nonhealing wounds.[26]

- The *American Academy of Orthopaedic Surgery* states: "Available data suggest that PRP may be valuable in enhancing soft tissue repair and wound healing."[27]

- A medical journal article from *Current Reviews of Musculoskeletal Medicine* states, "PRP provides a *promising alternative to surgery* by promoting safe and natural healing."[28]

- At a 2009 *International Cartilage Repair Society* medical meeting held in Miami, studies were presented that documented the efficacy of PRP therapy. The therapy was described as, "a promising method for treatment of cartilage defects."[29]

In PRP therapy, the patient's own blood is filtered and then placed in a centrifuge that rotates at high speed, separating the red blood cells from the platelets. The platelets—tiny cells within the blood that contain hundreds of growth and healing factors involved in the body's natural healing processes—are concentrated by the spinning into a PRP mixture. The PRP is then injected into arthritic joints or injured areas, such as the hip, knee, or shoulder. This high concentration of platelets—anywhere from three to ten times the concentration found in normal blood—stimulates the growth of new cartilage and tissue. PRP injections can heal torn ligaments and tendons, and even fractures that don't heal when treated by other measures! In the near future, higher concentrations of platelets may be possible. I have attended medical conferences where researchers have reported getting great results from concentrating the platelets sixteen times greater than found in normal blood.

PRP is loaded with approximately three hundred rejuvenative growth factors that encourage healing. Growth factors are just like they sound: factors within our own blood that promote tissue, cartilage, and bone growth. How handy is it that if you need the fibers of a torn body, tissue like a tendon or ligament—or even a broken bone—to heal? Very handy!

Many conditions respond to PRP therapy. They include injuries to the back, neck, jaw, elbows, shoulders, hands, hips, knees, ankles, and feet. Even diabetic and decubitus ulcers can respond to PRP measures! However, when the condition doesn't respond to PRP alone or when in my medical judgment they are needed, then stem-cell therapy—using stem cells that originate in an individual's own fatty tissue and bone marrow—can come to the rescue when PRP alone or other *Beyond the Knife* therapies aren't sufficient. In fact, I gather the stem cells from my patient's own fat cells by using a special liposuction blunt needle inserted into the fatty area near the belly button. This procedure is done under local anesthetic and is practically painless. I am using stem cells more and more, as I find that the combination provides the benefits of PRP with the exceptional healing benefits of stem cells. In my experience PRP is often even more effective when combined with ASCs.

Broader Uses of ASCs

Stem cells, "have been shown to support the health of the nervous system, cardiac function, liver function, pancreatic function, and kidney function as well as the lungs, skin and bones," states Christian Drapeau, MSc, in his book, *The Stem Cell Theory of Renewal: Demystifying the Most Dramatic Scientific Breakthrough of Our Times.*[30] In that book, he maintains that stem cells help maintain the health of the entire body:

The discovery that increasing the number of circulating stem cells equates to greater health … offers a new strategy in the pursuit of health and wellness.

Stem cells constitute the natural renewal system of the body … [this] has paved the way to a new paradigm in health and wellness … Every day of our lives, the role of stem cells is to patrol the body and migrate into areas needing assistance.[31]

Drapeau continues: "The number of stem cells circulating in the bloodstream has been shown to be a determinant factor for overall health. More stem cells circulating in the blood equates to greater health."[32] That's because more stem cells are available for the day-to-day natural repair processes throughout the entire body.

Therefore, the discovery of the natural renewal system of the body … open[s] the door to a novel way of looking at health. Instead of looking at health as an absence of illness and at any health-promoting strategy as a way to postpone illnesses, we can begin to look at health as a natural process, an intrinsic ability of the body to restore itself. The human body possesses the natural ability to remain healthy, and supporting this natural ability by increasing the number of circulating stem cells is logically the best way to enjoy optimal health.[33]

I agree with Drapeau's observation that increasing the number of circulating stem cells is logically the best way to enjoy optimal health.

Drapeau's observations were made before it was understood that ASCs can also be harvested from our own fat tissues. In my experience, Drapeau's comments also apply to MSCs from adipose tissue. Combined with PRP, those substances can successfully be used to treat patients with severe, as well as less severe, conditions.

Stem Cells for Better Human Performance

Beyond simply meeting the day-to-day wear and tear challenges of daily life, our bodies are challenged by strenuous activities, such as hiking in the mountains, competing in a triathlon, bike riding and/or exercise walking.

Like the exercise challenges just mentioned, over time, any physical activity beyond normal day-to-day activity creates small injuries in the bones, muscles, tendons, and ligaments of the body.

When the body needs to replenish its tissues to repair those injuries, as it does on a regular basis, stem cells in our bone marrow receive a chemical signal that activates them, causing them to migrate to the site of injury and initiate the process of cellular repair. However, as the body ages, the signal for this migration fades, the ASC population decreases and their ability to heal is diminished. That's when injections of MSCs are needed.

Keep in mind that MSCs are ASCs that can be harvested from bone marrow or adipose tissue. Regardless of whether they were harvested from bone marrow or from adipose tissue, they are pluripotent. They offer enormous potential for treating a wide range of diseases and disorders, including diabetes, heart disease, and musculoskeletal ailments, including cartilage and bone damaged by injury or osteoarthritis.

When MSCs are injected into an environment where there has been loss of or damage to cartilage, new cartilage cells, known as chondrocytes, form. When injected into collagen, new collagen secreting cells are the result. When injected into bone, they form osteoblasts, the basic building blocks of bone. Injected into torn vascular muscle cells, the MSCs cause the creation of new vascular muscle cells. MSCs can also turn into skin cells or even nerve cells. Furthermore, these ASCs can even turn into the body's most important muscle cells: heart cells.

What most people don't realize is that when they get a small tear in a tendon or ligament, the body heals the tear by forming scar tissue over it. This scar tissue is predisposed to recurrent symptoms, because it is not the same quality tendon as one that is uninjured. A tendon repaired naturally with scar tissue does not have the same resilience; it does not stretch and go back to its original size like an uninjured tendon does. Consequently, this lack of resilience may cause recurrent symptoms. Also, if a future tear should occur, it is likely to be larger, and the type of tear that people come to me to fix.

However, when PRP is given with stem cells, the stem cells are able to turn themselves into uninjured tendon cells. No weak spot remains. That's why I say stem cells and PRP can make tendons better than ever!

To fix such injuries, at present, surgeons use all sorts of surgical procedures, including arthroscopy with fracture chondroplasty. I predict that stem cells, either alone or in connection with a surgical procedure, will be used more frequently to help these patients. In fact, the use of stem cells to help healing in surgical procedures is worth a book of its own. However, since our title is *Beyond the Knife*, the uses of stem cells with surgery are beyond the scope of this book.

Uses of ASCs Combined with PRP in Orthopedics

ASCs, often combined with PRP, are finding new uses in my specialty: orthopedics. That's because PRPs, as pointed out in a previous chapter, are rich sources of growth factors. This is being noted worldwide.

Leading medical researchers in Poland write, "The use of growth factors in combination with tissue engineering seems to be the most promising method ... for the treatment of tissue, bone, and cartilage defect(s)."[34]

Cartilage is an interesting substance. For centuries, doctors have been frustrated by the inability of damaged cartilage to repair itself. This obstacle has limited the chance of a patient's complete recuperation from serious injuries that affect the ankles, knees, shoulders, and other major joints. This is especially problematic for knee injuries suffered by anyone under the age of forty-five.

The cartilage in the knee does not naturally regenerate in the body. That's because there is very little blood flow to the inside of the knee joint. All of the nutrition of the cartilage cells is obtained from the synovial fluid, secreted by the synovial membrane that encloses the joint. This leaves the cartilage cells very limited access to the stem cells available in circulating blood. This compromised circulation is why it is so important to add stem cells to the treatment of an arthritic joint.

— Regeneration of Broken Bones

The combination of PRP with stem cells is a superb way to stimulate bone growth, a therapeutic approach that is increasingly used in the treatment of complications of bone healing processes. PRP accelerates the bone regeneration process because, as previously explained, it is loaded with growth and healing factors.

Bone regeneration begins with the release of the growth factors PDGF, TGF beta 1, and IGF from PRP. It often takes six to eight weeks before results become apparent, but when it does, patients literally jump with joy. Instead of being crippled, they can walk, run, and even climb mountains!

The value of PRP and stem cells working together is demonstrated whenever they are used to repair tissue and bone.

In an interview with Dr. Breecher, my coauthor, one of my patients, David Robert, a Sunrise, Florida, appliance repairman, tells how the combination helped him in his fight against arthritis.

> When I went in to see Dr. Lazar, I couldn't raise my arms over my head. I now am able to reach over my head and grab

something down from a shelf because he injected stem cells into my shoulder joint. That's very important to me because I repair appliances. It's imperative that I be able to reach for things, especially when I am bending over a dishwasher or fixing something behind the electric range in a kitchen. I was in constant pain before having the PRP and stem-cell therapy treatments. Now, I can say that after the treatments, the pain isn't there anymore.

For me, that's what my medical practice is all about: helping patients heal themselves and conquer pain. PRP and stem cells are state-of-the-art tools that help me do just that. In fact, I predict that in the near future, medical doctors will be offering periodic IV injections of stem cells as the ultimate preventive medicine!

— Two Stem Cell Harvesting Techniques Available at My Office

We utilize mini-abdominal liposuction procedures to harvest ASCs from adipose tissues to use in fat graft applications. The adipose extraction procedure is similar to liposuction, which is used to slim and reshape the body. For bone marrow extraction, we turn to the iliac crest, which offers easy access and the most abundant source in the body. The iliac crest is the thick curved upper border of the ilium, the most prominent bone of the pelvis. You can feel the iliac crest by pushing your hands to the sides of your waist.

There are many more stem cells per cubic centimeter (cc) in the body's adipose tissue than in bone marrow. There are about 150,000–200,000 stem cells per cc. However, more total stem cells can be harvested from bone marrow. When a patient has a very serious problem, we may need to tap both sources to ensure enough stem cells for optimal treatment.

To approximate the harvest of the same quantity of stem cells that we get from fat tissue, we have to extract much more blood and concentrate from bone marrow than from adipose tissue. When we use our concentration process on adipose tissue, we are able to multiply 10 cc (from a healthy male) and turn that amount into two million available stem cells, a good amount with which to fix a knee joint. To get a similarly large quantity of stem cells from bone marrow, we have to do a larger extraction (60 cc) from the marrow. In a 60 cc bone marrow aspiration, there are as many as 50 million stem cells.

It is easier to harvest stem cells from a patient's fatty tissue than it to harvest from bone marrow of the iliac crest. It also is much less expensive to remove adipose stem cells than to remove stem cells from bone marrow. It is always best to harvest stem cells from a person's own fatty tissues when that source will be sufficient.

— Adipose Tissue Stem Cell Harvesting

Picture this: the patient is led to a comfortable-looking procedure room and asked to lie down on his back. I arrive in cap, gown, a mask over my nose and mouth, and sterile gloves on my hands.

The patient has been draped and prepped: that means the area where the fat is to be removed is scrubbed with a powerful germ killing liquid. The skin is numbed by a local anesthetic. An advantage of harvesting stem cells from fatty tissue is that the procedure does <u>not</u> require anesthesia or heavy sedation. Once numb, I make a small nick in the skin with a #14 gauge needle. That becomes the entryway for a special mini-liposuction needle.

The whole procedure is almost painless and takes less than an hour. I use a 10 cc syringe to infiltrate local anesthetic—a 50-50 mixture of Marcaine and Lidocaine—into the subcutaneous fat. We wait several minutes for the combination anesthetic to take effect and then 20 cc of sodium chloride is injected into the subcutaneous fat. Normal saline is then infiltrated into the fat, using an in and out motion to mix the fat with the saline for three minutes. After adding the saline, we again wait, this time for five minutes. Then, we insert another mini-liposuction needle attached to a 20 cc monoject syringe. Once inserted, we rock the needle using an in and out motion drawing out the subcutaneous fat-containing stem cells. We continue this process until the syringe is filled with about 40 cc of fat-containing stem cells, normal saline, and local anesthetic.

Immediately following the extraction procedure, the patient is again prepped with a sterilizing fluid, and a small two-by-two-inch dressing is applied. While this is being done, the syringe is inverted, needle side up, for about fifteen minutes, or until the fat cells separate from the stem cells. The fat and saline solution can now be discarded.

For the vast majority of cases, this adipose tissue stem cell harvest is sufficient to bring effective healing. But, it is nice to know that more help is available from stem-cell containing bone marrow. Again, the amount of stems cells needed depends on the severity of the case.

— Bone Marrow Stem-Cell Harvesting

Bone marrow stem cells (BMSCs) come from the iliac crest, the bony, thick, curved, upper borders of the ileum, the most prominent bone on the pelvis.

You can feel the iliac crest by pushing your hands on your sides at your waist, feeling for the bone and following it down and to the front.

To harvest the ASCs from that location, we have the patient lie on his or her side. We give a mild sedating anesthetic and then make a nick in the skin. That's so the needle used to extract the bone marrow does not traumatize the skin. Through that small hole, we insert the needle of the syringe through the iliac crest into the liquescent part of the bone and extract the stem-cell-containing bone marrow aspirate. The aspirate is then filtered for application in the most difficult cases.

Because they are *autologous* (that means from the patient's own body), like PRP, ASCs are safe. No blood diseases or viruses from other people can be transplanted.

The best news is that these autologous ASC injections often eliminate the need for surgery. According to an article in the *Journal* of *Current Medical Research and Opinions,* "At first these cells contribute to the growth of the organism by increasing the dimension of the organs then, after growth is completed, the main role of a stem cell is homeostatic."[35] "Homeostatic" means that ASCs renew and/or regenerate the cells of damaged tissues and then helps them maintain the internal equilibrium of the body part being treated.[36]

Are PRP and Stem-Cell Therapies Safe?

They certainly are.

For over twenty years, the application of autologous PRP has been safely used and documented in many fields of medicine, including cardiology,[37] orthopedics, sports medicine, dentistry, neurosurgery, ophthalmology, plastic surgery, urology, wound healing, and maxillofacial repair. Consequently, PRP is a well-studied treatment for conditions that have traditionally required surgery or other extensive treatments:

PRP and ASCs are derived from the patient's own body tissues and blood, so there is absolutely no risk of transmissible diseases such as hepatitis, HIV, West Nile fever, and Cruetzfeldt-Jakob disease (a variant of Mad Cow disease). There is also no chance of rejection by the patient's immune system. Nor can they cause hypersensitivity reactions.

Indeed, PRP has been used for over thirty years as an aid in recovery after surgery in many fields of medicine.

Stem cells have been used almost as long. Thousands of research articles have been published attesting to the safety of PRP and ASCs. Furthermore, there are countless case studies of individuals helped by PRP and ASCs, both in conjunction with surgery and for patients who desired nonsurgical treatment.

Take-Home Points from Chapter 2

- PRP and stem cells are state-of-the-art, modern healing tools.
- The combination of PRP and stem cells is a superb way to stimulate bone growth.
- Adult stem cells (ASCs) are harvested from the patient's own bone marrow and/or adipose tissues (fat cells).

3

State-of-the-Art *Beyond the Knife* Treatments Allow Faster Healing for Professional Athletes and Weekend Warriors

The guy who plays softball on weekends, the woman who runs a 5 km race every now and then, the avid golfer or tennis player—all often suffer common orthopedic injuries. These are some of the people for whom PRP therapy is ideal. That's because PRP can help them avoid surgeries that would have kept them from their athletic activities for months.

But remember, the effects of PRP are enhanced when combined with ASCs. Indeed, surgery is no longer necessary for many common athletic injuries. *Beyond the Knife* PRP therapy, combined with ASCs, is particularly effective in injuries from sports activities such as:

- Professional football knee injuries

- Tennis or golfer's elbow

- Pitcher's arm injury

- Hard-to-heal volleyball or softball shoulder injuries

- Other athletic injuries, including those to the knee or ankle

As an example, in 2009, football fans followed the tribulations of Hines Ward, wide receiver for the National Football League's Pittsburgh Steelers. He had injured his knee in the AFC playoffs and was in pain and limping. The injury was so serious it didn't look like he would be able to play in the Super Bowl.

His pain and limp came from a painful seriously sprained medial lateral ligament. Lateral ligament injuries usually take a minimum of eight weeks to as much as many months to heal. Yet, Ward did play in the Super Bowl and actually caught a winning pass thanks to PRP therapy. As we discovered in chapter 3, PRP is a therapeutic substance created by a simple process involving the centrifugation of the patient's own blood.

If you are struggling to heal a sports injury, and wondering if PRP might be a good choice for you, you may be asking, "Just how credible are the reports of success with this treatment?" Many positive reviews attest to its effective application for healing. Successful PRP treatments for athletic injuries are well documented at medical meetings and in the medical literature. Consider these findings:

- PRP releases a supra-maximal quantity of three hundred healing substances called growth factors that "stimulate recovery in non-healing tissues," according to an article in *Current Reviews of Musculoskeletal Medicine.*[38]

- "The use of biologically active factors currently holds great promise in the field of sports medicine," conclude the authors of a 2006 medical article.[39] That promise is now being met.

- "In recent years there have been rapid developments in the use of growth factors for the accelerated healing of injury," write the authors of a 2008 article in the *British Journal of Sports Medicine.*[40]

- At the International Conference on Regenerative Medicine, Dr. M. Sanchez and his colleagues reported on a case series of six athletes with Achilles tendon ruptures. PRP was applied to the ruptured Achilles tendons of these professional basketball and football players. The athletes who received an injection of PRP to the wounded ends of the tendons recovered their range of motion quicker. They experienced no wound complications (surgery would have created a wound) and "took less time to run and resume training."[41]

Many athletes, including pros and weekend warriors, have benefited from PRP. For example, Golf champion Tiger Woods has had several PRP procedures. PRP may have helped him continue his winning ways. At the 2010 press conference surrounding the Masters Golf Tournament, Tiger confirmed that he received four injections of PRP to treat a knee injury, a tear to his ACL ligament. He also confirmed receiving numerous treatments for recurring injuries to his Achilles tendon, injuries that adversely affected his lateral collateral ligament and, consequently, his ability to drive golf balls long distances. He told reporters that the treatments were successful, and "helped speed my recovery."[42]

Now we'll look a little closer at the application of PRP through the firsthand experiences of many of my patients. The following anecdotes are from real people and their stories are true. (By the way, the names of noncelebrity patients in this book have been changed to protect their privacy, unless they have given us permission to name and quote them. Many have.)

Injured Tennis Champion Is Able to Play at Championship Levels Again

Jill Sterling, a fifty-five-year-old champion tennis player from Plantation, Florida, suffered from excruciating tendonitis (tennis elbow). Jill's case got so bad that one time, she even had to walk off the court in tears, forfeiting a tournament. In anguish and in so much pain, she came to our office.

Many painful conditions, including tennis elbow, are resolved by just one or two injections. But, more complex conditions might respond more fully with additional injections of PRP. For Jill, this meant three injections. However, just four months after her very first treatment, Jill was back on the tennis courts, winning games. Each successive injection fostered additional strength and healing.

Jill is just one of hundreds of my patients who have been able to avoid surgery with less invasive alternative healing modalities like PRP.

Baseball Pitcher Is Able to Fire off His Best Pitch Again

Another of our patients is Michael Adams, a twenty-three-year-old baseball pitcher for the Franklin Pierce College baseball team. Michael is the son of Fred Adams, who played baseball professionally for the Detroit Tigers and New York Mets. Michael's dream is to follow in his father's footsteps and become a professional baseball player.

He has a good chance to obtain that dream, because he has a pitch that is a combination fastball and curveball (he calls it a "flyer") that helped him strike out forty-two batters in four games (33.2 innings) during the 2008 college baseball season. The year before, he led the Northeast College 10 League in innings pitched (112) and had eleven wins in fifteen starts.

His record was so good that he had hopes of being drafted by the Boston Red Sox once he graduated. However, that hope almost died in March 2009, when he threw the ball hard and, to use his words, "I heard a crack and felt a sharp pain, like something had just broken in my elbow. I couldn't finish the game the pain was so great," Michael told me.

The pain continued after the game and incapacitated him so much he couldn't even pick up anything with that hand, let alone throw a baseball. "I feared I would never play college baseball again, much less be drafted by the Boston Red Sox," Michael added.

His doctors prescribed physical therapy and corticosteroids and other anti-inflammatory agents for months, but he received no relief and had to stop playing baseball. For further treatment, Michael was referred to one of the team physicians for the Boston Red Sox. An MRI revealed he had torn the ulna collateral ligament of his right elbow. The Red Sox doctor treated him with PRP, but Michael experienced the procedure as extremely painful ("I almost jumped off the table," Michael said ruefully). The treatment worked only partially. Consequently, the team physician for the Red Sox referred Michael to our office.

When Michael came to see us, a follow-up MRI revealed a residual tear of the ulna collateral ligament at the point of the insertion of the long bone of the forearm (the ulna) into the right elbow. No wonder it was painful. We promised him he would feel no pain during the PRP treatment at our office. In July 2009, Michael received that treatment. "Dr. Lazar numbed my arm with anesthetic so well that this time I didn't even feel the needle go in. It was painless," Michael said.

The injection worked and, over time, healed the torn ligament. By September, Michael returned to college and once again was able to throw a baseball. Today, his hopes of being drafted by the Red Sox remain alive!

PRP Helps Photographer Resume Photography and Tennis

Thomas Martin, a fifty-four-year-old professional tennis instructor and photographer, also benefited by PRP therapy. He was referred to my office early in 2009 with a tear of the common flexor pronator tendon. The pain referred over to his elbow; it was another classic case of tennis elbow. In his case, it was so bad that the pain interfered with such activities of daily living as tying his shoe or even using an electric can opener. In January of 2009,

Martin arrived received a PRP treatment at our office. Within weeks, he was able to resume playing professional tennis and teaching and has had no recurrence of earlier symptoms.

Injured, Young, Softball and Volleyball Player Plays Again and Wins Scholarship

Take the case of M.C., a seventeen-year-old female softball and volleyball player. A few years earlier, she had injured her shoulder during a game and had not told her parents. (Advances in medical technology can now reveal injuries that often went unnoticed by medical personnel in earlier years.) Consequently, she had endured right shoulder pain for several years. During that time, she had difficulty throwing, hitting, or doing anything that involved the external rotation of her shoulder. Finally, her parents became aware of her condition. An MRI showed a labral tear. (That's an injury to the shoulder joint.) It's called a SLAP injury, because the injury is to the superior labrum, anterior (front) to the posterior (back) of the labrum. She was lucky that it was a small, minor labral tear. PRP was the answer for her bum shoulder. Unfortunately, neither PRP nor platelets can repair major labial tears.

Shoulder Anatomy

Let's look at some basic anatomy. The shoulder joint has three bones: the shoulder blade or scapula, the collarbone or clavicle, and the upper arm bone or humerus. The head of the upper arm bone (the humeral head) rests in a shallow socket in the shoulder blade. The humeral head is usually much larger than the socket, and a soft fibrous tissue rim called the labrum surrounds the socket to help stabilize the joint. If the labrum is torn, it doesn't do its job of stabilizing the joint. This typically results in inflammation and pain.

In the old days, surgery was the only answer. Doctors made an incision and stitched up the torn labrum. Now we can inject PRP with or without a combination of stems cells. We did add stem cells to our treatment of our seventeen-year-old patient, M.C. She not only successfully avoided surgery by receiving PRP/ASC therapy, but she has also been able to resume athletic activities so well she was awarded a college volleyball scholarship!

PRP Is an Accepted Therapy

One sports organization used to consider PRP "doping" (an illegal practice) wrote two researchers in a 2008 issue of the *British Journal of Sports Medicine*.[43]

In fact, as of 2009, PHP is no longer on the WADA list of prohibited substances.

Closer to home, the National Football league and Major League Baseball currently regard PRP and stem cells as medical treatments, not as performance-enhancement agents, so the use of those substances is left to the discretion of team physicians.

Pro athlete or weekend warrior, PRP, stem cells, and other *Beyond the Knife* alternative therapies may just be the best answer for you.

How Does PRP Work?

PRP is a concentrated blood sample of platelets. It usually contains four to five times the amount of platelets found naturally in our blood. Intensive research on PRP has led to the identification of substances called growth factors that initiate all human wound healing. Among the growth factors are:

- PDGF—(platelet-derived growth factor)

- TGFs (transforming growth factors)

- IGF (insulin-like growth factor)

- CTGF (connective tissue growth factor)

- EGF (epidermal growth factor)

- BFGF (basic fibroblast growth factor)

- VEGF (vascular endothelial growth factor)

Since this is not a book on biological science, we briefly discuss the first two of these growth factors and then we address the third, which is a "superfamily" of curative compounds. Healing injured tissue and bone in the body is a complex process involving four distinct phases. Each of these phases is coordinated by growth factor release and cell-to-cell interactions.

PDGF is the first growth factor to be released by PRP into a wound. It stimulates revascularization (the growth of new blood vessels), collagen synthesis (creation of new cartilage), and bone regeneration.

A second very important protein appearing in PRP is IGF. IGF is also a stimulator of bone formation.

The third factor, TGF, refers to a superfamily group of curative compounds that include bone morphogenetic proteins. BMPs have increasingly been used in clinical practice to encourage healing. Unfortunately, the cost of BMPs is very high, precluding wider use in everyday clinical practice. However, PRP contains an abundance of BMPs, so when PRP is being used, you get a bargain: you get BMPs as well as other healing substances within PRP, such as the cytokines interleukin-1 and interferon.

TGFs also contain TGF beta 1 and beta 2, which are basic growth and differentiation factors involved in the healing of connective tissue and bone regeneration. (Differentiation is the process by which cells or tissues change into a more specialized form or function. For instance, sometimes you need tissue cells, sometimes new collagen, and with bone fractures you need to encourage the growth of bone cells.)

PRP contains not only three hundred growth factors to do all this but also, "many biologically active substances including … about 2,000 proteins. Microbiological tests demonstrated activity of these peptides against disease causing microbes such *as Escherichia coli, Staphylococcus aureus, Candida albicans* and *Cryptococcus neoformans*," wrote a team of prestigious medical researchers.[44]

Furthermore, the investigators also pointed out that they observed antimicrobial activity of PRP against antibiotic resistant MSSA and MRSA Staphylococcus aureus, the virulent germs that are becoming resistant to standard antibiotics. Consequently, the antimicrobial effects of PRP may become even more valuable as scientists discover additional applications for their use. In other words, PRP doesn't just deliver a one-two punch. It delivers a one-, two-, three-, four-, five-, six-, and more "punch" of various curative substances that encourage cells—whether the cells are tissue, collagen, or bone cells—to repair themselves.

Each of the three factors has its own role to play, and together, they control and regulate your natural healing process. The PRP process concentrates these growth factors within platelets containing fibrin and stem cells so that each cubic millimeter of PRP solution contains 1.5 to 2 million platelets, resulting in a fivefold increase in bioactive growth factors. That's why the substance is called platelet rich plasma.

A robust, curative response is stimulated by concentrating these growth factors and injecting them at the site of an injury. Because it is so concentrated, PRP acts as a potent tissue growth stimulant by amplifying the natural process of tissue repair and healing. When the platelets are injected into injured areas, such as a damaged arthritic joint, PRP stimulates the growth of new cartilage. When injected into torn tendons or ligaments, new fibers grow and heal the tears. This regeneration shortens rehabilitation time and eliminates the need for surgery in many cases. In fact, I presently treat many elite college and some professional athletes for muscle, ligament, and tendon injuries. Athletes are a joy to treat, because they heal rapidly. They respond to the platelets and, most of the time, do not need stem cells. Still, stem cells are good for those with more severe injuries.

Let's Take a Quick Look at the PRP Procedure

Since the "shelf life" of the growth factors in PRP is not long, a maximum of about eight hours if anti-clotting measures are used, the healing growth factors become activated as soon as the PRP clots. Consequently, it is vital that your doctor take steps from the beginning of the platelet harvesting procedure to see that the blood from which PRP is taken, and the PRP itself, does not clot until the doctor is ready to apply it to the treatment site.

The patient has a role in ensuring successful harvesting of his or her PRP. One of the most important things for patients to do starting several days before the procedure is to drink a lot of water. The body has to be hydrated so blood flow is fluid enough to harvest the platelets. We recommend that patients drink eight to ten glasses of water in the twenty-four hours before their appointment. We tell them to avoid alcohol, coffee, tea, and soda pop prior to the procedure, as those substances can dehydrate your body.

Anti-inflammatory medications, such as Motrin, Nuprin, Ibuprofen, Aleve, Naprosyn, Celebrex, and Voltaren, should be avoided for four days before each injection and for two weeks after each injection. Those substances can interfere with the important growth factors contained in PRP. An alternative to those medications is NaturaCell, a facilitator of growth factors that enhances healing by encouraging the growth of stem cells in the body.

For Those Afraid of Needles, the Pain is Much Less than the Injury Needing Treatment

We use a special needle in the syringe used for platelet harvesting, because we don't want the platelets to be damaged in a regular syringe. If they were damaged, they would prematurely release the various growth factors that they contain.

The procedure itself takes place under local anesthesia in a special procedure room where we extract a minimal amount of the patient's blood. Using a sterile needle, the blood is taken from a large vein, such as the wrist vein (the cephalic vein) or the antecubital vein, the large vein on the inside of the elbow, which is the one that lab technicians (phlebotomists) usually use when taking blood for blood tests. However, we take much less blood.

Blood tends to coagulate (clot), so the syringe used to take the blood contains an anticoagulant substance: known as ACD-A. The harvested blood is then placed in a sterile container or test tubes and then centrifuged to produce the optimal PRP composition.

To separate and concentrate the platelets, the device must use two separate centrifugation formats, called spins. The first spin, known as the *separation spin,* separates the red blood cells from the rest of the whole blood—white blood cells, platelets, and plasma. It's this portion of the blood that is spun next. This is called the *concentration spin,* which separates and then compacts the platelets, white blood cells, and a small amount of remaining red blood cells. After 95 percent or more of the red blood cells have been removed, the remaining plasma is sequestered into another compartment of the receiving chamber.

The resulting fluid still contains a few residual red blood cells and nearly all of the white blood cells and platelets. Because it is compacted, heavy, and dense, it accumulates at the bottom (the PRP compartment of the receiving chamber). This accumulation is overlaid by a volume of plasma that floats on top of it. These blood components are separated by a thin white line, called the "buffy coat," that separates the PRP from the mostly clear or yellow liquid that rises to the top. This yellow fluid is platelet *poor* plasma (PPP) and is discarded.

The remaining red blood cells accumulated at the bottom are commonly described as the *red blood cell button.* It is created by the presence of younger, more complete platelets that contain concentrated growth factors. This red suspension is the PRP used to treat the patient.

The newly developed PRP is anticoagulated. That means it is clot free and will remain in that state until the clotting process is initiated. PRP can remain sterile and its platelets remain viable and bioactive for up to eight hours when stored at room temperature. However, PRP is most effective when we use it on the patient's injury almost immediately. Of course, the site of the patient's injury is totally numbed by anesthetic prior to injection of the PRP.

The clotting process can be initiated by adding thrombin or calcium. We have found just the right amount of thrombin and calcium to add to the PRP. However, we often don't have to initiate the clotting process, because it occurs naturally when we inject the PRP into ligaments, tendons, and muscles. When I inject the PRP, I use a state-of-the-art ultrasound machine to diagnose the condition and perform ultrasound guided injections to see where the sterile needle must be inserted and where the freshly harvested platelets and growth factors must go in and around the injured site. Clotting takes place quickly, as the healing growth factors are immediately released into the site of the patient's injury.

Another Reason PRP Is Safe and Effective

It's very safe and effective. A state-of-the-art ultrasound machine assures that the PRP is inserted in the proper places to heal the injury. And remember: PRP is derived from the patient's own blood, so there is no risk of rejection or disease transmission. This helps ensure the procedure's safety.

As for effectiveness, patients usually obtain 50 percent relief of their pain from the first injection. On the second injection, relief of 80 percent to 100 percent is often obtained. PRP has been used for over thirty years to aid in recovery after surgery in many different fields of medicine. There are thousands of research articles published on the safety of PRP. There are countless case studies of individuals helped by PRP, both in conjunction with surgery and those who desired nonsurgical treatment.

In the following chapters, you'll learn more about what conditions PRP can heal, especially in conjunction with ASCs. You will also hear from other patients who have experienced that healing and of other alternative *Beyond the Knife* therapeutic remedies.

Take-Home Points from Chapter 3

- PRP and ASCs can be wonderful therapies for many patients with chronic tendinosis, acute muscle and tendon tears, and many other orthopedic injuries that plague both professional athletics and weekend warriors.

- Young or old, PRP is often the very best answer to athletic orthopedic injuries.

4

PRP and Stem-Cell Therapies to Heal Arthritic Joints

At age sixty, David Robert, of Sunrise, Florida, was afraid he would have to retire early. Osteoarthritic pain in both shoulders was interfering with his ability to work and enjoy life.

"I have almost no range of motion in my arms or shoulders. I can't lift my arms up straight in front of me, much less get something down from a top shelf," he told me. Besides having difficulty lifting, pushing, and carrying, to cope with the severe pain in his shoulders, other doctors had put him on anti-inflammatory prescription drugs and narcotics. "Have you ever tried to repair a toaster while under the influence of a narcotic?" he asked me. "It would take me two or three times as long to finish a job as it used to. The shoulder pain was so bad I couldn't sleep on either side because of the pressure and pain. I had to sleep on my back."

We diagnosed his problem as osteoarthritis, combined with a torn rotator cuff in each shoulder. Other doctors had recommended surgery on both shoulders. Surgery has been the unequivocal standardized treatment for torn rotator cuffs, and it takes many months of rehabilitation to heal from that surgery. However, from my thirty years of surgical experience, I knew that surgical repair wouldn't work on his severe injuries. So, we took him off the narcotics and anti-inflammatory medications and administered several injections of PRP, guided by our ultrasound device. The results were amazing! We saw his pain levels decrease by 50 percent as a result of PRP therapy.

Next, we used stem-cell treatments, again guided by ultrasound, for both the osteoarthritic areas of his shoulders and both torn rotator cuffs.

"I am now able to reach above my head, and I can work comfortably," he reports. "I am off all pain medications and am more productive. I can now lie on either side and sleep comfortably."

Osteoarthritis

Osteoarthritis is by far the most common type of arthritis—an estimated 27 million Americans ages twenty-five and older have osteoarthritis, according to the National Institute of Arthritis and Musculoskeletal and Skin Diseases.[45]

Arthritic joints, like those Mr. Robert had, can be caused by osteoarthritis, also known as degenerative joint disease. Osteoarthritis occurs when the cartilage that cushions joints breaks down. Without the cushioning effect of cartilage, bone rubs against bone, which causes pain and stiffness. It happens most frequently in the knees but can also affect the hips, fingers, neck, and toes.

Being overweight or obese is far and away the biggest risk factor for developing osteoarthritis. One study analyzed 316 obese adults who underwent a diet with and without specialized exercise. This eighteen-month study compared the effects of exercise alone, dietary weight loss alone, and a combination of exercise plus weight loss. The study concluded that a combination of exercise and dietary weight loss resulted in improved mobility and pain reduction.[46]

Rheumatoid Arthritis

Another form of arthritis is rheumatoid arthritis (RA). According to a study by the World Health Organization, musculoskeletal injuries are the most common cause of severe long-term pain and disability, affecting millions of people worldwide.[47] While, bone and cartilage injuries extract a high financial toll in loss of income and the expense of remedial treatments, musculoskeletal conditions, including osteoarthritis, cost nearly $128 billion per year in direct medical expenses for loss of income and productivity and for surgical procedures such as total joint replacements.[48] Osteoarthritis medicines, for instance, accounted for an astronomical $5.31 billion of US household medical expenditures in 2007![49]

RA is an autoimmune disease ("auto" means self), so-called because a person's immune system, which normally helps protect the body from infection and disease, attacks itself for unknown reasons. RA most frequently attacks joints, causing debilitating pain and inflammation.

A joint is any junction in the body where two bones meet. Ligaments connect bones, and cartilage acts like a shock absorber between two bones. If the cartilage starts to break down, bone rubs against bone. The result: pain and stiffness of osteoarthritis or RA.

The joint is also surrounded by a ligament-like structure called a capsule which protects and supports it. Remember, a joint capsule is lined with a type of tissue called synovium, which produces synovial fluid, a clear substance that lubricates and nourishes the cartilage and the bones inside the joint capsule.

When RA strikes, the synovia becomes inflamed, causing uncomfortable warmth, redness, swelling, and pain. During the inflammatory process, the normally thin synovia becomes thick, puffy, and sensitive to touch. As the disease progresses, the inflammation spreads from the synovia to damage the cartilage and bones of the joint. This progressive disease also affects and weakens surrounding muscles, ligaments, and tendons. During this autoimmune process, people with RA suffer severe chronic pain.

The pain can lead to other illnesses. Severe, chronic RA pain, accompanied by progressive joint destruction, disability, and disfigurement, is known to increase the risk of experiencing emotional disturbances, such as depression. Patients with RA are twice as likely to be depressed as people in the general population.[50]

Treatment Options

Many treatment solutions have been developed to enhance tissue regeneration and reduce the adverse effects of inflammation and other degenerative arthritic mechanisms. Oral autoimmune medications are the mainstay of treatments by rheumatologists. Other treatments found to be useful include changes in diet, intra-articular injections, and physical therapy/rehabilitation.

In my office, we use PRP and ASCs, which have proven to be a combination that contain a powerhouse of healing factors that moderate the inflammation while healing the underlying causes.

Diet and moderate specific exercises are especially beneficial to obese people with arthritis. Many medical studies have indicated that losing excess weight puts less stress on the joints and helps prevent further osteoarthritic injury. Furthermore, vegetarian diets have been shown to decrease the synovial inflammation caused by the auto-immune process associated with arthritis.

Vegetables in the nightshade family—such tomatoes, potatoes, eggplant, and most peppers—are notorious for causing inflammation, especially in people with osteoarthritis. Ronenn Roubenoff, MD, a nutritionist at Tufts University School of Medicine, says this occurs in up to 2 percent of all patients with arthritis.[51] Make sure you are not in the unlucky 2 percent, because if nightshade vegetables do not cause you ill health, there is no need to avoid them. In fact, for most of us, they provide health benefits. Nightshade vegetables provide a number of health benefits, because they are typically rich in vitamins, minerals, and other healthy compounds. For instance, tomatoes are a good source of lycopene, a phytochemical thought to have antioxidant effects that may protect against cancer. Spicy peppers boost your metabolism and, thus, help you lose excess weight.

However, if you are among the minority who feel worse after eating nightshade vegetables, you would probably be better off by eliminating or reducing your intake of nightshades.

Avoid exercise that causes the feet to hit the ground with high impact, thereby putting added stress on weight-bearing joints. This can make osteoarthritis worse. So, avoid running, playing basketball, or tennis, because those sports are likely to exacerbate symptoms and accelerate the progression of osteoarthritis. Instead, try exercises like cycling, swimming, and using a rowing or elliptical training machine to strengthen muscles (including your heart), which place little or no stress on the joints.

Another way to help reduce stress on arthritic knees is to wear shoes that provide good support. Wearing special shoes and using orthotics within the shoes are very important measures to prevent osteoarthritic injuries. They provide support, especially shock absorption. Check with a podiatrist to see if orthotic inserts to your shoes will help.

When Diet and Exercise are not Enough, PRP, or PRP with ACSs, May Be the Answer

Unfortunately, diet and exercise alone just don't do the job for many people. If these two approaches fail to provide satisfactory results, the most promising nonsurgical treatment is PRP alone or a combination of PRP with stem-cell therapy.

Medical researchers have reported remarkable results using PRP in the treatment of osteoarthritis of the thumbs, knees, and hips. The medical literature also reports on the success of PRP in resolving painful RA of hips, knees, and shoulder joints, resulting in the patients experiencing less pain and enjoying improved range of motion.

Used alone, medical researchers have reported remarkable results using PRP in the treatment of common injuries, including the regeneration of bone and cartilage, and when treating osteoarthritis of the thumbs, knees, and hips. Indeed, the medical literature is full of reports on the resolution of painful osteoarthritis of hips, knees, and shoulders resulting in patients enjoying improved range of motion.

However, I am now getting better results using a combination of PRP and ASCs from two sources within the patient's own body. My protocol for severe OA-caused problems is guided ultrasound PRP and ASCs from bone marrow aspiration concentrate (BMAC) followed approximately four weeks later with another PRP procedure, depending on the patient's condition, either with or without a fat graft containing ASCs from adipose tissue. For less advanced OA two PRP/fat grafts four weeks apart may be all that is necessary although sometimes additional injections are needed.

When PRP and stem cells guided by ultrasound are injected into injured areas, such as an arthritic joint in which the cartilage has been damaged, the PRP/ASC combination stimulates the growth of new cartilage. New fibers actually sprout and grow, reinforcing the joint or sealing and healing the tiny tears in tendons or ligaments. This regeneration shortens rehabilitation time and eliminates the need for surgery.

There are surgical procedures used to repair cartilage. A good surgeon can harvest cartilage from a place in your body where you don't need all of it and transplant it to where you do need it—to your knee, for instance. However, in my experience, these surgical operations are short to intermediate in terms of their effectiveness. But we now have a better option. We can go *Beyond the Knife* and use the PRP/ASC combination.

The lack of natural regenerative ability of the cartilage in the knee joint is due to its limited access to stem cells. PRP alone doesn't attract enough stem cells to generate the therapeutic response needed for healing to take place. We overcome this problem by providing the joint with ASCs, along with the PRP.

When Stem-cell therapy Is Necessary

In arthritic joint conditions, especially advanced arthritic conditions, we might even start with stem-cell therapy. In advanced arthritic joint conditions, the cartilage has almost completely been destroyed. The damage caused by osteoarthritis, for example, is often too serious to be healed by PRP alone. That's why I started using stem-cell therapy for those cases. Stem cells stimulate the growth of new cartilage and can actually turn themselves into new cartilage.

Remember, Mesenchymal stem cells (MSCs) are multi-potent cells that can transform into a variety of cell types during the body's tissue repair process. Cell types that MSCs have been shown to differentiate into include collagen-secreting cells, bone-forming osteoblasts, and cartilage-forming chondrocytes.

These characteristics make MSCs an ideal candidate cell type for tissue-engineering efforts aimed at regenerating replacement tissues for diseased structures. Either through direct cell-to-cell interaction or their secretion of various healing and/or growth factors, MSCs can exert a tremendous effect on local tissue repair.[52]

Those ASCs are present in multiple locations in the body, but they are most easily extracted from stomach fat. As mentioned earlier, I harvest those stem cells using a mini-liposuction device. Almost all patients love receiving this bonus of decreasing their stomach fat!

For several years, I was one of only a few physicians in the world using fat-derived stem cells to treat successfully joint injuries caused by osteoarthritis.

MSCs have been used successfully in many medical fields, including orthopedic, maxillofacial, cosmetic, spinal, and general wound healing, so it just seemed natural for us to try stem-cell therapy for our patients with osteoarthritis. This is called an *autologous mesenchymal transplant,* and it, too, often eliminates the need for surgery.

Take-Home Points from Chapter 4

- Diet and moderate, specific exercises are especially beneficial to obese people with arthritis.

- A vegetarian diet decreases inflammation experienced by rheumatoid arthritis patients.

5

Nonsurgical Treatments for Joints, Tendons, Ligaments, Shoulders, Elbows, and Knees

The use of PRP and stem cells in my practice are powerful therapeutic modalities to treat muscle, tendon, and ligament injuries. Stem-cell therapy is already adding another dimension to healing for those with joint injuries.

PRP and stem-cell therapy guided by ultrasound have helped patients who couldn't even perform the activities of daily living resume their normal lives. Our new patients tell us:

- "I'm having trouble lifting my baby grandson."

- "I am having trouble lifting my groceries from the cart and placing them into the car."

- "I'm stiff when I wake up."

- "I can't walk for very long periods of time."

- "I can't sit for very long. When I sit too long, I have difficulty getting up because I am so stiff, and it hurts me."

These are common complaints of patients who come to our office for treatment and have been helped by PRP or other *Beyond the Knife* therapies, including stem cells.

Injured body locations most likely to be helped by PRP include knees, elbows, shoulders, hips, backs, joints and their connective tissues, tendons, and ligaments. As mentioned previously, a joint is where two bones meet. A joint may be immovable (fibrous), as those of the skull; slightly movable (cartilaginous), as those connecting the vertebrae; or freely movable (synovial), as those of the elbow and knee. It is among our synovial joints that a complex of bones, ligaments, cartilage, and tendons come together. Arthritic joints occur when there is loss of or damage to cartilage. The damage causes the joints to lose their ability to absorb shock, resulting in inflammation and pain.

Tendons are composed of collagen fibers. They connect muscles to bones, making everyday physical motions and activities possible. Tendons are inelastic and strong and occur in various thicknesses and lengths. Without the ability of tendons to connect to bone, it would be impossible for the body to walk, run, jump, lift, carry, and do other important actions of movement.

The spectrum of tendon injuries ranges from acute tendonitis (associated with increased physical activity) to chronic tendinitis (chronic degeneration of the tendon) and may be exacerbated by age-related degeneration of the tendon. Overuse or damage to the tendon over a long period causes the collagen-based fibers in the tendons to form small tears. That's the condition known as tendonitis. That type of tendon damage most often occurs in the knee, ankle, shoulder, wrist, bicep, and Achilles tendons.

Ligaments are also composed of collagen fibers. They attach and hold one bone to another, stabilizing joints and controlling range of motion. Ligaments differ from tendons in that ligaments are the fibrous, slightly stretchy connective tissues that bind joints together and connect bones and cartilage. Ligaments control the range of motion of a joint and stabilize the joint so bones move in what we consider proper ways. For instance, your elbow can't bend backward. When a ligament is damaged, it is no longer able to provide support, and the joint is weakened and may become painful.

PRP and stem-cell therapy guided by ultrasound are good for patients who aren't helped by conservative therapies (rest, ice, compression, elevation, and cortisone injections) and thus face surgery because of their injuries. It is thought that PRP initially inhibits excess inflammation, while stimulating the spread and maturation of cells within the injured area.[53]

By using ultrasound to make pinpoint injections where they are most needed, we have successfully treated patients with PRP who have had pain in their joints, muscles, and ligaments located in many "trigger points" and even some diagnosed with fibromyalgia, a condition identified with abnormal neurotransmitters. Patients with fibromyalgia often don't get better with other treatments. However, we have successfully treated several of these patients with two or more injections of PRP, and the results were astonishing. Every one of them got better.

Because PRP comes from the patient's own blood and is used right away, it has an excellent record of success and safety. For instance, one of our fibromyalgia patients was a young tennis player who had suffered pain for ten years and had tried every possible therapy and treatment. We treated her with PRP, and she now raves about how great she feels, not only on the tennis court, but all the time.

If you suffer from arthritis, an injured ligament or tendon, and traditional methods have not provided relief, PRP or PRP combined with stem-cell therapy may be your solution. These procedures are less invasive and less expensive than even the most conservative surgery. They can heal tissue with minimal or no scarring and alleviate further degeneration of the tissues. Surgery cannot do that.

During surgery, tissues surrounding the injured site are damaged by the surgical incision, and there is always scarring. Alternatively, many injuries can be and are healed with just one or two simple PRP/stem-cell injections.

Humans are unique individuals, and responses to treatment vary. Most patients are helped by one or two injections of PRP and stem cells. Patients with more serious diagnoses may require as many as three injections given four to six weeks apart. The results depend on the quantity and quality of the patient's own stem-cell and platelet growth factors. The risks and side effects of PRP and stem cells are minimal and do not increase with the number of injections. And remember: since the stem cells and PRP are harvested from the patient's own body, there is no chance of disease transmissions from donors.[54]

Let's look at some of the body locations that can be helped by PRP and then look at some case histories from my files.

The Shoulder—Joints, Tendons, and Ligaments

PRP and stem-cell therapy are most useful in treating parts of the body that tend to get injured as we get older. They include the shoulders, elbows, knees, hips, and ankles, are usually responsive to PRP/ASC treatments. A commonality of all these body sites is that soft tissues and bones are connected together by cartilage, tendons, and ligaments that provide support and guidance for these various joints. These joints, and the connective soft tissues and bones, are prone to injury through accident or simply through aging and the accumulated built-up stresses of living.

The shoulder is one of God's greatest masterpieces. Consider how the shoulder is used and the fact that most people take it for granted. There is more movement in the shoulder joint than any other in the body. The shoulder can assume about sixteen hundred positions. The shoulder is truly a remarkable creation.

That is, until something goes wrong. The shoulder joint is composed of three bones (the shoulder blade; the upper arm bone, or humerus; and the collarbone, or clavicle) and four joints: the acromioclavicular (AC) joint, the glenohumeral (GH) joint, the scapulothoracic (ST) joint, and the sternoclavicular (SC) joint.

The AC joint is a common site for the development of osteoarthritis in middle age. The GH joint is the most susceptible to injury, because it is entirely dependent on non-bony connections to hold it in place. The GH joint relies on the balance, strength, and control of muscles, tendons, ligaments, and cartilage to function properly.

One of the sites within the shoulder that tends to become injured is the rotator cuff. The rotator cuff (rotor cuff) is the group of muscles and their tendons that stabilize the shoulder. When there is a tear in the rotator cuff—or in muscles, ligaments, or cartilage elsewhere in the body—pain and stiffness frequently result and can be treated by PRP and stem cells.

However, if the pain is caused by a more advanced and painful rotator cuff condition called impingement, we can't treat it effectively with PRP or stem cells, because it is an anatomical condition that probably needs surgery. (We go *Beyond the Knife* when we can. Unfortunately, there are still reasons for surgery.)

Impingement occurs when the top bone called the Acromion—or the CA ligament attached to it—rubs against the rotator cuff or the bursa that pads the cuff. This occurs from overuse, osteoarthritis, or overactivity. Consequently, a spur from the clavicle or the acromion (the bony crest covering the rotator cuff) rubs like a spike against the cuff and the bursa, which is a closed, fluid-filled sac that provides a gliding surface to reduce friction between the different parts of the rotator cuff. The over activity of stressful tennis serves, for example, can damage your rotator cuff and its supporting ligaments, creating a tear. In response, the acromion produces additional bone to support the damaged ligament. The resulting bony spur takes up space between the acromion and the rotator cuff, causing the pain of impingement when it rubs against the cuff and its bursa. The tear in the ligament can be treated by PRP and stem cells, but the bony spike often has to be removed surgically.

Remember sixty-year-old David Robert, the owner of the appliance repair company in Sunrise, Florida? He had a torn rotator cuff. He is one of many who had shoulder problems that responded well to a combination of PRP and stem-cell therapies. He told one of our associates the following:

"When I went in to see Dr. Lazar, I couldn't raise my arms over my head. I now am able to reach over my head and grab something down from a shelf. I repair appliances. It's imperative that I be able to reach for things, especially when I am bending over a dishwasher or fixing something behind an electric range in a kitchen. I was in constant pain before the PRP and stem-cell therapy treatments. The pain isn't there anymore. I am so glad I found Dr. Lazar."

Another patient, whom we will identify only as B.C., had shoulder surgery. But, months after the surgery, she still had difficulty moving, lifting, carrying, bending, and moving her shoulder. Besides the surgery, she had been treated with oral anti-inflammatories, analgesics, rest, physical therapy, and muscle stretching and strengthening exercises, all to no avail. However, she then was treated with several PRP injections to her right shoulder and has responded nicely to them. She has had approximately 70 percent relief of her symptomatology and is now able to move, lift, carry, bend, and use her arm in a more comfortable manner.

Another happy PRP shoulder repair patient is Star Eugene, forty-three, who works as a deputy sheriff for Miami/Dade County. In 1991, she was injured while working in a home for developmentally handicapped adults.

> I was helping one of my patients out of the shower when I slipped. I tried to catch her and prevent her from falling, but she fell on top of me. My shoulder hit the tile floor. The fall tore some tendons and ligaments in my shoulder. I felt a sharp pain.
>
> After the accident, I couldn't even lift a pan of water without pain. I had limited range of motion in my right shoulder. It became a Workman's Compensation case, and I wasn't able to have surgery until 1995. It didn't work so well, and eleven years later, in 2006, I had to go under the knife again. However, my pain and weakness persisted. It was excruciating. I was taking one hundred eighty pain pills every month to cope.
>
> Dr. Lazar told me about PRP in 2008, and I said I would try anything.
>
> We did the PRP. I had two shots last year and two shots this year. My arm is at least 85 to 90 percent better. I am now able to go to the gym, and I am able to lift things the way I used to. I am a police officer, and I need that shoulder for my job.
>
> The PRP injection site was painful for a short while at

the time of the injection, but it has been so worth it. The amount of relief I have received from this procedure is just phenomenal.

Dr. Lazar is my savior. He is my angel.

Let's look at another body site that often can be helped by PRP.

The Elbow

A condition called elbow epicondylitis (elbow tendinitis) is a common problem for people whose jobs or other activities require strong gripping or repetitive wrist movements. While it can affect almost anyone's "funny bone," the condition can be especially excruciating for athletes. When it occurs in athletes, the condition is popularly given the name of the person's sport. For instance, "tennis elbow," "pitcher's elbow," and "golfer's elbow" are terms used to define these injuries. The only difference between tennis elbow and golfer's elbow is that with tennis elbow, the damage is done to the extensor carpi radialis on the outside of the elbow. With golfer's elbow, the damage is typically on the inside of the elbow, to the flexor carpi radialis, a muscle in the forearm that flexes and moves the hand.

Patients with these conditions often complain of severe, burning pain on the outside part of their elbow. The pain can be made worse by gripping or lifting objects. Lifting even small, light objects, such as a book or cup of coffee, can lead to significant discomfort. In severe cases, the pain can radiate to the forearm.

The condition is usually caused by a tear in one of the tendons that extend from the elbow to the wrist and fingers. It is typically minor and usually resolves with non-operative treatments, such as rest, ice, compression, and elevation. However, in some cases, those nonsurgical approaches fail, and patients come to me looking for an alternative to what, in the past, was the next step: surgery. Sometimes tennis elbow is resistant to such conservative treatments because it can be caused by nerve compression. However, it too responds to PRP.

Golfer's elbow is another example of this type of injury. The injury often happens when a golfer, during a swing off the tee, hits the ground and the ball at the same time, gouging a piece of turf from the green. This is normal, but sometimes the golfer's stroke makes a divot that is too large or hits a rock or a tree root. If this is done too often, or if the golfer is playing with clubs that fit poorly and do not help absorb the shock, the resulting impact is transmitted to the inside of the elbow, stressing the flexor tendon. An accumulation of such shocks can tear the flexor tendon.

Another common example of this type of injury is called pitcher's elbow. It occurs in the elbow's ulnar collateral ligament and results from the violent external rotation of the pitcher's windup and throw.

As mentioned, when these conditions did not resolve after rest, icing, hot pads, anti-inflammatory medications, bracing, and/or physical therapy in the past, the next step was surgery. Now, the next step can be PRP or a combination of PRP with ASCs.

The use of PRP has been studied scientifically in this type of condition. A California colleague and his assistant, physical therapist Terri Pavelko, studied 140 patients with elbow epicondylar pain. All patients had persistent pain extending for periods longer than three months. Twenty patients met the study's criteria. Five were controls, and fifteen patients were treated by PRP. (Three out of the five controls dropped out of the study to seek PRP treatment intervention.)

These PRP-treated patients were examined four weeks, eight weeks, and six months after the PRP treatments. Within four weeks, the PRP-treated patients reported their elbow pain had improved by a mean of 42 percent. Eight weeks after treatment, they reported a mean of 60 percent reduction in pain. At six months, the PRP-treated patients had improved their pain scores by 81 percent.

Twenty-five months after the treatment, 91 percent of the patients reported "complete satisfaction" with PRP. The other 9 percent reported some degree of continuing pain. The 91 percent were able to return to their activities of daily living.[55]

The authors concluded that the PRP-treated patients had, "demonstrated significant improvement with a single injection that was sustained over time with no reported complications."[56]

My own elbow tendinitis patients also rave about PRP. Take, for example, Donald Saunders, a sixty-four-year-old Plantation, Florida, man who presented at our office not only with lateral epicondylitis and osteoarthritis of both elbows but also a torn meniscus in his knee. He had difficulty lifting, carrying, bending, and reaching. His knee problem caused him difficulties in bending, squatting, lifting, carrying, and stair walking. He described his condition and treatment:

> I'm an old fat guy with gray hair. About two years ago, I decided to start pumping iron again. After about a month, I added more weight and did more repetitions, and I kept getting sorer and sorer. It got so bad that I couldn't even pick up a small set of dumb-bells weighing only five pounds. I couldn't lift a chair and move it from one side of the breakfast

table to the other. I would be afraid to pick something up, because I feared I would drop it. When I tried to pull the cord to start the lawn mower, it hurt for about three days afterward. After PRP, now it doesn't hurt at all!

Dr. Lazar explained that I had an accumulation of injuries and torn tendons that had not healed. "Doc" Lazar took some of my own blood—a small amount compared to what I give at the blood donor center every fifty-two days—and he injected the platelets from my own blood into the sore spots below my elbow joints. The injections were relatively painless. I've had cortisone shots in the past that hurt more.

It took about six weeks for the healing effect to be felt, but now I am able to pick up and carry anything I want to pick up. Now when I want to mow the lawn, I don't have to worry about pulling the rope to start the lawn mower. Now it doesn't hurt at all.

When asked if he felt the PRP procedure was painful, he answered, "No, it didn't bother me at all. The platelet-harvesting portion was like giving blood to the Red Cross. I think PRP is a marvelous procedure. It's wonderful that PRP stimulates the body to heal itself."

Another of our happy elbow patients is Tom Mindenhall, a fifty-four-year-old photographer and tennis teaching professional who had a tear in the elbow's flexor pronator tendon. The pain was so severe he had to quit playing tennis at the professional level. The pain had progressed to the point where he had pain just doing normal everyday activities. After PRP, Tom is back in the game.

The Knee

Knee injuries can bring pain, disruption to one's life, and cause a lot of frustration. Does your knee click, lock, or give way? You might have a tear in the meniscus. There are actually two menisci: crescent-shaped pads of cartilage present in each knee. The menisci improve knee function by spreading your weight across the joint, improving joint stability, and helping to circulate synovial fluid around the knee.

The menisci can be easily injured by the force of rotating the knee while bearing weight. The pad on the inner side of the knee is the medial meniscus and the one most likely to suffer damage. The only blood circulation to the meniscus is to the outer one-third of the meniscus pad, and, thus, the rest of that part of the knee is susceptible to injury. A partial or total tear may occur when a person quickly twists or rotates the upper leg while the foot stays put (for example, when turning to hit a tennis ball). Menisci injuries are fairly common.

Typical signs of a menisci tear include swelling and difficulty moving through the full range of knee motion. Another symptom includes pain on rising after you squat. Sometimes, a mobile segment of torn menisci lodges in the knee joint, and you may feel frequent locking of your knee or be unable to fully extend your leg. Meniscus tears can take many shapes: Vertical, horizontal, "parrot beak and "bucket handle" shapes are just a few.

One of our first PRP patients was Sandailo Saiz, seventy-nine, who suffered from severe osteoarthritis. When he first came to see us, he explained he had suffered from chronic pain inside his knee for about a year. The pain interfered with his ability to walk.

His case demonstrates the effectiveness of PRP over traditional methods. Before starting to use PRP, the traditional treatment was an injection of hyaluronic acid, a natural substance found in the knee joint, followed by an injection of cortisone. The patient was then advised to apply ice to the injured area for fifteen minutes as often as possible.

That's the treatment Mr. Saiz received during his first visit. However, he still had inflammation and pain in his knee a month later. Once again, he was treated with cortisone, told to use ice, and advised to get physical therapy for a month.

The third month, he saw us again, and his knee was getting worse. A buildup of fluid had occurred. We used a needle procedure to remove the fluid in his knee and again administered a shot of cortisone.

He came back the fourth month and reported that he still had difficulty walking. By that time, our office had some early experience with PRP. This time, we injected 10 cc of PRP from his own blood. Success! Four weeks later, he returned to my office, completely asymptomatic. This time, his knee looked normal. There was no buildup of fluids. He had no pain, and wasn't taking any pain relievers or anti-inflammatory medications. He told us the outcome was like a miracle to him.

Another of our star patients is Joshua Mislow, a twenty-six-year-old Fort Lauderdale plumber who had an injury to his right knee in July 2006. He came to see us because he had persistent symptomatology. He had difficulty bending, squatting, walking, and getting up from a sitting to a standing position. He was in constant pain.

I will let Joshua explain his situation.

I tore the medial meniscus in my right knee so severely that I had to have surgery. I had two surgeries before PRP was used. The operations were done by doctors other than Dr. Lazar. The surgeries actually made the injury worse. I was completely dependent on painkillers for over two years just to be able to be semi-functional. I couldn't walk and I couldn't work.

Amazingly, after two simple PRP treatments, I have almost 100 percent resolution of the pain. The only time my knee feels uncomfortable now is when it rains in the summertime. Then I get a few twinges.

I am now a normal person. I have been able to return to work full time as a plumber, and that involves a lot of climbing, squatting, crawling, going up ladders, and even working upside down in hard to reach places. I couldn't do any of these things anymore before I had the PRP treatments.

Still another of my successful PRP knee patients is Rena McMunn, a sixty-four-year-old retired hairdresser from Margate, Florida. Speaking of PRP, she said, "It's fabulous. It [PRP] took away the pain right away. It worked beautifully. Before PRP, it was difficult to walk. I couldn't even get out of my bed and walk into the dining room. Now I can pretty much do anything."

PRP and stem-cell therapies are revolutionary treatments. There are also revolutionary treatments in the fields of complementary and alternative medicine. They are the subject of the next chapter.

Take-Home Points from Chapter 5

- The body sites that PRP and ASCs therapy are most useful in treating are those that tend to get injured as we get older. They include the shoulders, elbows, knees, hips, and ankles.

- Joints, tendons, and ligaments can also be successfully treated by PRP and ASC therapies.

6

Complementary and Alternative Medicine Options to Surgery

One of the best things a physician can do for his or her patients is to help them combine the best of traditional medicine with the best of well-researched alternative and complementary therapies. The object is to heal the body using the least stressful means that work.

Complementary and alternative forms of medicine (CAM) therapies are thought of as "holistic," because they focus on the whole body rather than separate body parts like Western medicine does. CAM therapies have assumed significant importance to patients with all types of ills, and for some patients, their application has helped them entirely avoid the need for surgery.

Almost four out of ten adults (approximately 38 percent) used some form of CAM to promote health and wellness or to treat a variety of diseases and conditions, according to the 2007 National Health Interview Survey.[57] According to the US government's National Center for Complementary and Alternative Medicine, Americans spent $33.9 billion out-of-pocket on CAM therapies.[58] Studies have shown that the most common conditions for which persons seek alternative therapies are neck (57 percent) and back (47.6 percent) problems.[59]

"Generally, persons who choose CAM approaches are seeking ways to improve their health and well-being or to relieve symptoms associated with chronic, even terminal illnesses or the side effects of conventional treatments. Other reasons for choosing to use CAM include belief in a holistic health philosophy, having a transformational experience that changes one's world view, and/or the desire to have greater control over one's own health," wrote the authors of a statistical report on CAM that was commissioned by the CDC and the National Center for Health Statistics.[60]

Since so many Americans use CAM therapies, it behooves us to understand what CAM therapies are and to identify those that might help you enhance health and perhaps allow you to avoid surgery for certain conditions.

Differences between Alternative and Conventional Therapies

Alternative therapies are defined as any treatment that is used instead of conventional medical treatment. Conventional medical treatment for many medical conditions includes the use of medicines (sometimes many types), radiation therapies, and various forms of surgery. These therapies are the cornerstones of modern evidence-based medical care and are often successful, even lifesaving, forms of treatment.

However, these cornerstone conventional approaches are also associated with side effects and adverse reactions, and people are afraid of experiencing those consequences. That's why there is a need for better *Beyond the Knife* therapies.

For reasons varying from cost to accessibility, to fear of prescription drugs, radiation, and surgery, CAM therapies have assumed significant importance to patients with all types of ills, especially cancer. The traditional approaches to cancer therapy have been surgery, radiotherapy, and chemotherapy. Those three modalities are the cornerstones in the management of most malignancies. However, those conventional approaches have associated toxicities and suffer from limitations in curing advanced malignant lesions.[61]

That's why some individuals suffering from cancer turn to CAM therapies. Certain CAM therapies have proved to be useful complementary treatments for cancer. For instance, traditional Chinese medicine (TCM), "has been used to treat colorectal cancer over the last 6,000 years or so with some degree of success," according to noted Asian researchers.[62] TCM has also successfully provided support for cancer patients undergoing radiation therapy.[63] In fact, it may even enhance the effects of radiation therapy, and since surgery sometimes follows radiation treatment, TCM may potentially reduce or eliminate the need for surgery in such cases.

Besides TCM, complementary medicine includes any diagnosis, treatment, and/or preventive measures that complement mainstream medicine by satisfying a need or demand not met by orthodox medicine. Here's an example of such a need. Cancer has been a battle fought on many fronts.

Besides radiation, chemotherapy is an accepted and often lifesaving type of cancer treatment. However, although modern-day chemotherapy can often save someone's life, they can also result in increased levels of fatigue, anxiety, and depression, with consequently detrimental effects on physical and mental function. This results in the deterioration of many patients' quality of life (QoL).

Complementary medicine has emerged in part because of the adverse and unwanted results that result from the use of traditional therapies in the treatment of cancer patients. CAM has made significant inroads as an accessory modality, because it provides complementary options that can create an improvement in general well-being, palliation (relief of pain and discomfort), and occasionally even promote remission of malignant tumors.

On the other hand, if not used wisely and with the knowledge of your physician, you could make things a lot worse for yourself. I strongly warn readers that if a medical doctor has diagnosed you with a life-threatening form of cancer, do not allow CAM treatments to delay you from seeking conventional medical help.

I also advise you to discuss with your medical doctor any complementary or alternative medical therapies you may already be using or be thinking of using. However, for that discussion, do look for someone who is open-minded and has a track record for working with various types of healers. You want to find a medical doctor who admits he or she is limited to certain treatments, recognizes those limitations, and is willing to refer you to other types of health professionals. The doctor might say, "There are eight other health-care professionals who complement my treatments. I will refer you to the best one for you." That "best" one might be an oncologist recommending chemotherapy, or it might be a CAM healer.

Dangers of CAM Therapies

While some CAM therapies may qualify as *Beyond the Knife* therapies, not all are equal. In fact, some CAM therapies can be dangerous. For instance, herbal therapy has a long history of being helpful, but in certain situations, it can be dangerous. For instance, if you absolutely, definitely have to have surgery, stay away from commonly used herbal medications such as echinacea, ephedra, garlic, ginkgo, ginseng, kava, st. john's wort, and valerian. They can cause serious problems, such as increased bleeding in patients during and after surgery.

Furthermore, individuals with diabetes need to be aware that garlic, ginger, and ginseng may affect blood sugar control. Likewise, people with hypertension (high blood pressure) would be wise to avoid licorice, because it may lead to increased fluid retention. Someone taking heparin (an anticoagulant), could find that goldenseal works against the drug's blood-thinning action. Conversely, garlic can increase the activity of warfarin (Coumadin), another anticoagulant.

Certain herbs can also increase or decrease the effectiveness of anesthetics, cause organ transplant rejection, and interfere with other medications. What it boils down to is that there are some CAM treatments with the potential to contribute to negative interactions when combined with traditional medicine. You have to do your homework and find out about potential herbal interactions if you plan to try herbal therapy. And, be sure to let your doctor know what herbal therapies you use.

Now, let's look at evidence that various alternative medical systems may work well enough to be considered *Beyond the Knife* therapies. Let's first look at a type of treatment that seems to have evolved away from its roots, possibly in a better direction.

— *HOMEOPATHY*

What is called "homeopathy" today in most instances is not. That's because the central core of homeopathy as it was originally practiced involved two core principles:

The *principle of similars*, that "like cures like"— diseases can be treated by a substance that produces similar symptoms in healthy individuals.

The *principle of dilutions* (or "laws of minimum dose")—the *lower* the dose of medication, the *greater* its effectiveness. Carried to an extreme, serial dilution can be carried out to the point where hardly any of the molecules of the original treatment substance remain.

Those were the original principles of homeopathy. However, today, a lot of healers call their treatments "homeopathic" just because they use microscopic amounts of multiple herbal elements to treat medical ailments. As a result of the microscopic herbal components, the definition of "homeopathic" in the twenty-first century seems to have evolved to encompass herbal treatments. However, these modern homeopathic healers do not seek to re-create the symptoms of the illness, and they are not all involved in serial dilution. Consequently, those modern homeopathic healers are not really following the old-fashioned core principles of homeopathy. They are actually seeking to treat the underlying cause of certain conditions with the healing properties of herbs. Indeed, herbal treatments have been considered beneficial by healers for thousands of years.

I know people gain relief from at least one homeopathic remedy, because I discovered a homeopathic medicine called traumeel, which I use followed by single platelet injections to control inflammation. I began using it so individuals like college and professional athletes can return to their athletic activity as quickly as possible. It had worked so well on those types of cases that I now use it on everyone I treat with PRP and/or stem-cell therapy.

Traumeel has herbal roots. It is composed of twelve botanical and two mineral substances. Herbal remedies like traumeel are botanical preparations with a rich history of thousands of years of use by shamans and medicine men. Many of our modern medicines have evolved from herbal use. For instance, the bark of the willow tree contains a natural form of aspirin that has been used for hundreds of years for pain relief.

So, I'm not disparaging all so-called homeopathic remedies, especially those that are herb based. Be warned, though, that there is no agreed-upon method of standardization for herbs and their content. Thus, care has to be taken to identify and use only those herbal elements that have a proven track record. Furthermore, care should be taken to make sure one buys from reputable sources who sell herbal preparations that are standardized, tested, and properly labeled.

To sum up, I use traumeel with great success. I also recommend the use of certain herbs, like ginger root and turmeric extract, in combination with other substances in several antioxidant and anti-inflammatory supplement preparations. I discuss this topic in depth in the next chapter.

– AYURVEDA

Ayurvedic medicine originated in India more than two thousand years ago. The underlying belief is that when any of the three humors of the body— known as *vata, pitta,* and *kapha*—become faulty or spoiled; they invade the muscle tissue and produce swellings (arbuda). These swellings infiltrate deep into the body and increase in size. There are three types of arbudas: raktararbuda (leukemia), mamsarbuda (soft tissue myoma), and adayarbuda (metastatic tumors).[64]

Ayurvedic therapy includes recommendations for a healthy lifestyle, using specific foods and herbs believed to be helpful not only in preventing the progression of diseases but also in making the patients feel better and more comfortable. Among the foods and herbs most highly recommended are Allium sativa (garlic) and Allium cepa (onion), which have been reported to have various health benefits, including protection against cancer, probably because both contain selenium, a cancer fighter.[65] Bacopa monniera also known as water hyssop, moneywort, or brahmi) has been reported to strengthen mental faculties and help manage insomnia due to stress.[66]

I have had personal experience prescribing an ayurvedic medicine containing ashwagandha, which is a natural anti-inflammatory. It has helped many of my patients.

However, in spite of the promise shown by some of these substances, consumers have to be cautious. Some of the drugs made using so-called ayurvedic formulas have been criticized and come under scrutiny by government health agencies because of reports they contain harmful levels of lead, mercury, and/or arsenic.[67]

Also, be aware that Indian medical literature has many case reports of "cures" of various ills through the use of ayurvedic therapies. However, there are no long-term scientific studies that show ayurvedic medicine is a preventive against surgery in any particular disease, except in the sense that the ayurvedic recommendations for a healthy lifestyle prevent the progression of various disease states and so, in that sense, may prevent or forestall surgery.

— TRADITIONAL CHINESE MEDICINE

TCM consists of a wide range of techniques, including acupuncture, electro acupuncture, herbal medicine, and pharmacology.

Various studies have shown, "favorable results … in the use of TCM either alone or in combination with chemotherapy to treat advanced colorectal cancer. The problem, at least in western eyes, is that 'most of the known reports of success are unfortunately based on case studies conducted on small numbers of patients'".[68] Nevertheless, "TCM represents a ray of hope for patients who suffer from advanced disease and many patients have already taken to it with anecdotal good results."[69]

Herbal preparations are often used in TCM. For instance, in a prospective randomized trial with 188 nasopharyngeal carcinoma patients, Chinese doctors studied the effects of cancer "destagnation" therapy by using an herbal formula consisting of *Astralgi membranaceus, Paeoniae rubrae, Semen persica and Carthami tinctorii* in combination with radiation therapy. In that study, ninety patients were allotted to the destagnation group (radiation plus destagnation) and ninety-eight to the control group (radiation only). The combined treatment group showed a, "statistically significant improvement in local control and overall survival," wrote the authors.[70]

➤ *The Concept of Qi*

The gulf between traditional Japanese and TCM and Western medicine is wide. Western medicine depends on identifying the causes of disease or dysfunction and eliminating them. Traditional medical philosophies from the

Orient believe good health depends on the flow of "Qi" (an invisible energy) along hypothesized channels or meridians of the body.

Meridians are thought to be the pathways through which positive and negative energies communicate between parts of the human body. For thousands of years, Oriental healers have believed that Qi is the most fundamental substance in the human body and is necessary for the maintenance of life activities. In fact, TCM holds that Qi, "is the most basic building block of the world."[71]

The Qi of the human body takes two forms. The first is coagulated Qi, which manifests as various structural components of the body, such as viscera, body figure, sense organs, blood, and body fluids. The second is diffused Qi, which manifests as the energy and life force that flows in the body but takes no concrete form. This energy is thought to flow within a fixed network of twelve invisible pathways or meridians. This is the most important concept of Chinese medicine. Western medicine has nothing like it. Indeed, Western medical researchers have been unable to find proof that those meridians even exist. They do not correspond to nerve pathways already identified and traced by modern medical researchers.

Nevertheless, Chinese doctors believe that Qi promotes the growth and development of the body and the distribution and discharge of blood and body fluids. Qi also has the functions of warming, defense, and homeostasis (keeping the body in balance). Wellness is achieved when opposite and complementary forces, called yin (feminine—cool, moist, nutritive, quiet) and yang (masculine—warm, dry, energetic, active) are in balance and promote the unobstructed flow of Qi.

All treatments aim to balance a person's Qi, because an imbalance of Qi, yin, and yang are believed to result in sickness. A broad variety of therapies and lifestyle enhancements are used to promote, maintain, and restore Qi. These include the use of herbal remedies for nourishment, acupuncture, acupressure, electro acupuncture, moxibustion (heat therapy created by burning a small, spongy herb known as mugwort), diet, massage, meditation, and exercises such as qigong and tai chi.

➤ *Acupuncture and Acupressure*

Practitioners of acupuncture believe they can manipulate Qi. They view acupuncture points as corresponding to physiological and anatomical features, such as peripheral nerve junctions.

Along the meridians lie specific acupuncture points. These points are connections between the positive and negative meridians and functions of the body, including internal organs and muscles. Chinese medicine has charted some five hundred such points, which have been used for centuries to treat ailments of the human body. These meridians are classified as yin or yang, depending on the direction in which they flow on the surface of the body.[72]

Although Western medicine has been unable to locate or trace the meridians, it has confirmed certain positive results of acupuncture. For instance, a phase II clinical study involving 183 cancer patients treated with acupuncture reported a 47 percent reduction in pain experience.[73]

A randomized, control trial suggested that simple finger acupressure at the P6 acupuncture point can decrease nausea and vomiting in cancer patients.[74]

In May 2010, a large study was published in the journal *Autonomic Neuroscience* that demonstrated why and how acupuncture and acupressure works. In science speak, the authors of the study wrote, "Several classes of molecules, such as neurotransmitters, cytokines and growth factors, have also been identified as possible mediators for specific acupuncture effects."[75] What that means it they believe acupuncture actually affects the neurotransmitters between the nerves and results in pain relief.

In July 2010, the results of a large study were announced, showing that acupuncture, as well as other CAM therapies such as transcranial magnetic stimulation and phototherapy, helped pregnant women who developed depression beat their disease. This was an important finding, because many pregnant women chose not to take antidepressant drugs for fear they will harm their babies.[76]

Why do I share all this with you? When people enjoy relief from pain, nausea, vomiting, and depression, they are much less apt to receive surgical interventions.

➤ *Acupuncture Has Helped Many of Dr. Lazar's Patients*

Acupuncture has been a successful CAM treatment for many of our patients. Indeed, over the years, we have had many patients scheduled for surgery, but because of the pain they were suffering, we first referred them for acupuncture for temporary pain relief.

To our initial surprise, some of those patients found their pain so relieved they were able to cancel surgery! Acupuncture sometimes helps symptoms by stimulating the body's own pain modulators, so that's why I sometimes recommend its use prior to surgery. It is the least invasive treatment.

However, the effects of acupuncture are so variable that acupuncture helped one of my patients with impingement syndrome in one shoulder but didn't help at all when impingement later occurred in his other shoulder! Consider this unusual case. A patient came to see me complaining of painful impingement syndrome problem in the rotator cuff of his left shoulder. He looked familiar, so I asked, "Didn't I see you last year for your right shoulder?"

He answered, "Yes. Don't you remember you referred me to an acupuncturist? Those acupuncture treatments gave me so much pain relief; the tear in my ligaments had time to heal itself."

I asked, "So, why are you back?"

"Well, now I have the same type of excruciating pain in my left shoulder. Naturally, I tried acupuncture again, but this time it is not working, so, here I am."

He had a torn rotator cuff, that combination of muscles, ligaments, and tendons in the ball of the shoulder joint. The rotator cuff is an important part of the shoulder, because it allows us to contract our muscles and move our shoulder joints. Instead of scheduling him for surgery, we scheduled him for treatment with PRP therapy. This made all the difference in the world. We fully expected PRP to help him, and it did.

Once he got pain relief from the acupuncture treatment on the right shoulder, the patient didn't want, or need, surgery on that shoulder. Months have passed, and he hasn't had to return for additional therapy on that shoulder.

However, acupuncture didn't work on his left shoulder. We needed to progress to the next level of treatment, the use of PRP, and we did. He is doing fine now and has been able to avoid surgery.

Many potential surgical candidates may need to look more closely at how the energy of their body affects their wellness and consider how certain energy therapies, such as acupuncture, might be applied as potential alternatives to surgery.

➤ *Tai Chi*

Tai chi is a mind–body practice used in Asian cultures for centuries to improve wellness and reduce stress. It is a moderate form of exercise that may be an effective therapy for improving health-related QoL issues and personal self-esteem. These factors are particularly important to individuals with cancer.

In a study by Mustian and colleagues,[77] women diagnosed with breast cancer, who had completed treatment within the previous thirty months, were randomized to receive twelve weeks of tai chi or conventional psychological and social support. After twelve weeks of therapy, the tai chi group had significant improvements in health-related QoL scores, in contrast to the group that received only the conventional psychological and social support, which showed declines in the QoL scores.

What's that got to do with avoiding surgery? Patients with poor QoL scores have been shown to be more likely to have their cancers recur and, thus, have to submit to further cancer treatments, including surgery.

— REIKI

Reiki is a Japanese technique for stress reduction and relaxation that also promotes healing. It is based on the idea that the unseen life force (Qi) energy flows through us and is what causes us to be alive. According to Reiki practitioners, when one's life force energy is low, one is more likely to get sick or feel stressed. If it is high, one is more capable of being happy and healthy.

Reiki is a Japanese word denoting "universal Life Energy." The discipline is based on the belief that when spiritual energy is channeled through the body's seven primary energy centers (called chakras) by a Reiki practitioner, the patient's spirit is healed. That in turn heals the physical body.

Usually the Reiki procedure is conducted with the client lying down or sitting in a chair fully clothed. The Reiki practitioner "moves" the client's own life energy called Ki around by making arm and hand movements above the client. Reiki has been used to counteract pain, fatigue, and anxiety.

Indeed, in one study of twenty-four cancer patients, participants in Reiki experienced improved pain control and improved QoL.[78] Another study was conducted of sixteen patients (thirteen female). The majority had colorectal cancer, and the remainder had other painful conditions that drained their energy. Before the research study on Reiki, all sixteen patients took a test to quantify their fatigue. At the end of the study, the participants again rated their fatigue levels. Those who received the Reiki treatments showed decreased levels of fatigue, so presumably, they were better able to fight off the recurrence of cancer.[79]

Cautions about CAM Therapies

CAM therapies are a grab bag of ancient medicines, physical techniques, herbal use, and body–mind approaches. "While some techniques show considerable promise, others seem to be outright inefficacious."[80] Yet, as we have shown, there is plenty of evidence (unfortunately, not all acceptable to Western eyes because of small sample size) certain CAM therapies, such as TCM and Japanese medicine, can be defined as *Beyond the Knife* treatments.

Nevertheless, individuals should not allow the use of CAM treatments to delay them from seeking conventional medical help. It is always best to discuss your condition with a medical doctor, especially in regard to any CAM therapies one may be using or considering using.

Take-Home Points from Chapter 6

- One of the best things a physician can do for his or her patients is to help them combine the best of traditional medicine with the best of well-researched CAM therapies. The object is to heal the body using the least stressful means that work.

- Studies have shown that the most common conditions for which persons seek alternative therapies are neck (57 percent) and back (47.6 percent) problems.

7

The Role of Supplements in Combating Inflammation and Preventing Surgery

If you have joint pain, stiffness, loss of joint function, and swelling that is warm to the touch, you may be the victim of inflammation.

Inflammation is a natural process in which the body produces white blood cells to protect us from infection. Everybody who has had a sore throat, rash, hives, or a sprained ankle or wrist has experienced inflammation that is beneficial. That type of inflammation is good because it enhances healing. The initial inflammation at the site of an injury represents our body's natural response to protect the injured part from further injury and bring additional healing factors to the area.

However, in far too many cases—in diseases such as arthritis, diabetes, gout, lupus, heart disease, and cancer—the body's immune system inappropriately continues to trigger the inflammatory response. Inflammation then becomes a villain, causing joint-destroying rheumatoid arthritis, shoulder tendonitis, gouty arthritis, and other painful diseases of the musculoskeletal system, including osteoarthritis, fibromyalgia, and low back, shoulder, and neck pain.

Hidden inflammation is also at the root of many chronic diseases, including heart disease, obesity, diabetes, dementia, depression, and cancer. It is this hidden inflammation that slowly destroys our internal organs and joints and, thus, interferes with our ability to function optimally.

Almost every modern disease is caused or affected by inflammation in the body. In the past, uncontrolled inflammation has led to the operating room and the stress of surgery because of the damage unchecked inflammation causes to our joints and organs.

In our modern society, inflammation is often treated with anti-inflammatory drugs, such as ibuprofen or aspirin, or even with prescription drugs, including steroids like prednisone. In fact, according to an article in the *American Journal of Medicine,* just as many people die from taking anti-inflammatory drugs every year as those who die from asthma or leukemia.[81]

There is a better way: the *Beyond the Knife* formulated supplement way. It makes use of natural substances, including antioxidants and enzymes that have proven useful for centuries in treating individuals whose immune systems are challenged by destructive inflammatory responses. Antioxidants are great moderators of inflammation.

Ideal formulations of supplemental vitamins, minerals, herbs, and enzymes can offer protection and treatment for our bodies against this rampant inflammation. In my opinion, one of the most important nutritional breakthroughs to happen in the years leading to the twenty-first century was the recognition that potent antioxidants are also anti-inflammatories. That's why the French and Italians are so healthy and live so long: they imbibe a lot of antioxidants in their red wine and from the olive oil they put on and in their foods.

For at least thirty years, various nutritional constituents have been embraced for their role in promoting optimal health and reducing the risk of chronic diseases. Basic research and human studies have demonstrated the power of micronutrients—vitamins, minerals, herbal blends, and enzymes— to promote health beyond simply preventing or remedying deficiency diseases. However, over the past decade, there has been a concerted campaign that debunks the importance of antioxidants and certain other supplements.

It is not the purpose of this chapter to add fuel to that controversy by defending specific supplements. However, when we consider some of the conflicting evidence, as expressed through these reports, the question arises: are we viewing the results of logical, accurate, objective contrasts, or are there sources of bias that skew the results? In my opinion, many of the new debunking studies are flawed, because they were done on sick or dying patients, for short durations, and with low-quality synthetic ingredients instead of high-quality organic ones.

Supplements do work. In fact, there was a study published in the peer-reviewed *Nutrition Journal* that reveals people who used multiple supplements for the past twenty years were in overall better health than both nonsupplement users and individuals who only consumed a single multivitamin/mineral supplement. Dietary supplements consumed on a daily basis by more than 50 percent of the 278 multiple supplement users included a multivitamin/

mineral, B-complex, vitamin C, carotenoids, vitamin E, calcium with vitamin D, omega-3 fatty acids, flavonoids, lecithin, alfalfa, coenzyme Q10 with resveratrol, glucosamine, and a herbal immune supplement. The majority of women also consumed gamma linolenic acid and a probiotic supplement whereas men also consumed zinc, garlic, saw palmetto and a soy protein supplement.

"Greater degree of supplement use was associated with favorable concentrations of serum homocysteine, C-reactive protein, high-density lipoprotein cholesterol, and triglycerides as well as lower risk of prevalent elevated blood pressure and diabetes," wrote the authors. [82] They explained that the results were all markers of good health. The participants were recruited in 2005 from a repeat customer list of Shaklee Corporation. The participants were asked to fill out an online survey that asked about fifty-five different Shaklee products. four hundred thirty-five of 1200 individuals successfully completed online questionnaires. However the second part of the study involved physical exams and lab tests. Only 235 of the participants attended a national meeting of Shaklee product consumers where they submitted to a twelve-hour fast and the necessary lab tests and physical examinations.

It was a wonderful well designed and well carried out study, an excellent piece of scientific research that showed that supplement usage does improve health. I am not alone in believing supplements work. A 2009 study in *Nutrition Journal* described an online survey administered in October 2007 to 900 physicians and 277 nurses. The health professionals were asked whether they personally used dietary supplements and their reasons for doing so. They were also asked if they recommend dietary supplements to their patients. The Healthcare Professionals Impact Study (HCP Impact Study) found that 72 percent of physicians and 59 percent of nurses make regular use of dietary supplements. The most common reason given for using dietary supplements was for overall health and wellness (40 percent of the physicians and 48 percent of the nurses). Furthermore, when asked whether they, "ever recommend dietary supplements to their patients," 79 percent of physicians and 82 percent of nurses said they did![83]

With that auspicious information presented, let me now focus on formulations of ingredients in supplements that battle inflammation and provide other health benefit that I recommend.

The Role of Supplements in Avoiding Surgery

The role of the carefully formulated supplements I have developed is to prevent and modulate inflammation in the body and, thus, help you avoid unnecessary surgery. I have developed two separate anti-inflammatory formulas: one that features essential antioxidants and another that features enzymes. Each formulation includes vitamins, minerals, herbs, and enzymes that support metabolism, but in different amounts and combinations designed to work together in synthesis to boost your body's healing systems. While each ingredient has its own health benefits, in combination with the other ingredients, their effect becomes synergistic. That means these nutritional constituents work together, and the power of the *combination* is greater than the individual components working alone.

The following is an overview of the ingredients of the two formulations. But remember: the importance of the ingredients is not just their power to impact inflammation individually. The importance is that the synergy between the components boosts their anti-inflammatory power, thereby protecting your body from future damage and resulting surgeries.

One formulation is my Natural Anti-Inflammatory Complex. It is composed of the antioxidants vitamin C and resveratrol, along with a proprietary blend of glucosamine sulfate, chondroitin sulfate, MSM, hyaluronic acid, boswellia extract, curcumin (from turmeric extract), green tea extract, and mixed bioflavonoids. There is a special enzyme blend of bromelain, serratiopeptidase, papain, chymotrypsin, ginger root, and omega 3 fish oils, as well as the minerals zinc, copper, and manganese. The exact formulation and specific amounts of these ingredients are proprietary information and, as of the writing this book, negotiations with a natural supplement manufacturer are under way to produce the formulation. By the time you read this, the product may be in production. If you like, you can Google my name for the latest news or write my office and request further information.

Here are the ingredients and some of the reasons they are included in this formulation.

— Resveratrol

Resveratrol, a substance found in red wine, possesses diverse biochemical and physiological actions including, "antiplatelet and anti-inflammatory properties."[84]

"The cardio protective ability of resveratrol stemmed from epidemiological studies indicating that mild-to-moderate alcohol consumption is associated with reduced incidence of morbidity and mortality from coronary heart disease," wrote the authors citing the seminal research that brought that finding to light.[85]

Besides being an anti-inflammatory agent, Resveratrol is also a potent antioxidant and has been found to induce angiogenesis, the growth of new blood vessels. In research studies, resveratrol has been shown to protect the cells of the heart, kidney, and brain. It has also been shown to prevent bone loss and improve the health and the life spans of experimental animals, and it is hoped that it does the same for humans.[86]

— Vitamin C, Zinc, Copper, and Manganese

These substances are "magic wands" that enable our bodies to produce enzymes, hormones, and other substances essential for proper growth and development. Vitamin C and manganese both facilitate the absorption of chondroitin and glucosamine. Zinc, copper, and manganese are called *micronutrients*, because they are needed in the body in only minuscule amounts. Yet, as tiny as these amounts are, the consequences of their absence are severe. For instance, an inadequate amount of zinc in the diet is speculated to be a primary risk factor for pneumonia in the elderly.

— Glucosamine and Chondroitin

Medical colleagues who are familiar with my work credit me with being the first doctor to put glucosamine and chondroitin together in a bottle. Now it is used extensively to promote joint flexibility. Glucosamine is involved in the formation of the nails, skin, tendons, eyes, bones, ligaments, and heart valves. It is found in high concentrations in joint structures. Glucosamine and chondroitin sulfate are components of articular cartilage, the smooth, glistening, white tissue covering the surface of most joints in the human body.

Articular cartilage facilitates the movement of one bone against another, because it has an incredibly low coefficient of friction that, coupled with its ability to bear very large compressive loads, makes it ideally suitable for placement in joints, such as the knee and hip.

The very complex composition and architecture of articular cartilage permits it to achieve and maintain proper biomechanical joint function over the majority of a human life span. It is composed mainly of water (70 to 80 percent by wet weight), collagen (a connective substance), and glucosamine.

Although many studies have shown that glucosamine and chondroitin alleviate arthritis pain and other symptoms, especially in injured joints, a National Institutes of Health (NIH) Glucosamine/Chondroitin Arthritis Intervention Trial (GAIT)[87] found the beneficial effects of glucosamine and chondroitin were no better than those found with a placebo. However, interpreting those results is complicated because participants taking placebo had a smaller loss of cartilage, or joint space width, than predicted. Furthermore, an earlier analysis of GAIT found that a subgroup of study participants with moderate-to-severe pain showed "significant relief with the combined supplements.[88]

No matter how long GAIT goes on, it is just one study. In over three hundred studies and twenty clinical trials, glucosamine has been proven to build joint cartilage. It can also reduce the destruction of cartilage and relieve depression caused by taking NSAIDs, which are commonly prescribed for people with arthritis. Glucosamine should be taken in conjunction with chondroitin sulfate for an even greater effect on osteoarthritis. It is available as a supplement, in the form of glucosamine sulfate, which helps to combat the causes and symptoms of osteoarthritis.[89]

As mentioned, I have recommended the combination to our patients for years. I was a pioneer in identifying the beneficial effects and recommending this combination to our patients. Many years of experience with the two substances has convinced me that glucosamine and chondroitin are beneficial, especially in protecting joints.

Hold the presses! This just came to my attention as this book was going to press. New data from the GAIT trial shows that those who took glucosamine and chondroitin for knee osteoarthritis pain had pain outcomes similar to those who took the expensive pain medication celecoxib.[90]

— MSN and Hyaluronic Acid

Discovered in 1980, MSM is an organic form of sulfur found in most foods. Although found in many raw foods, including meat, fish, certain fruits, vegetables, and grains, it is destroyed when foods are processed or cooked, making supplementation necessary.

MSN is beneficial to healthy connective tissues because it:

- Helps maintain circulation throughout the body

- Supports healthy joints

- Maintains structure of proteins

- Strengthens connective tissues

Hyaluronic acid (HA) is a natural, cementing and protective substance that forms a gel in the intercellular spaces of the knee.[91] HA is also in the vitreous humor of the eye, as well as in other moveable joints. Intra-articular HA treatment for osteoarthritis of the knee was approved by the US Food and Drug Administration (FDA) in 1997, after it was researched and found to be used successfully in the treatment of inflammation in osteoarthritis of the knee. In comparison with NSAIDs and corticosteroids, the better tolerability and fewer adverse effects of HA have made its use widely accepted in recent decades.

— Boswellia Extract

Another powerful ingredient in this anti-inflammatory formula is boswellia extract. The first report in scientific literature of the, "novel anti-inflammatory properties," of the herb boswellia frereana was published on November 25, 2009, in *Phytotherapy Research*, while this book was being written. It was titled, "*Boswellia* frereana (frankincense) suppresses cytokine-induced matrix metalloproteinase expression and production of pro-inflammatory molecules in articular cartilage." [92]

Boswellia frereana is the frankincense mentioned in the New Testament as one of the gifts to the Baby Jesus carried by the three kings from the Orient. The herb was studied in the Connective Tissue Biology Laboratories of Cardiff University in the United Kingdom.

The researchers found boswellia, "prevents collagen degradation and inhibits the production of pro-inflammatory mediators," indicating its effectiveness as a therapy for treating osteoarthritis. The researchers said that, "due to its efficacy," boswellia should be further examined as a, "therapeutic agent for treating the inflammatory symptoms associated with arthritis."[93]

Having learned of the anti-inflammatory properties of boswellia several years ago, we have included it in our anti-inflammatory formulas, which have helped many of our patients keep their conditions from worsening and, thereby, eliminating their need for surgery.

— Turmeric

We have also added turmeric to this anti-inflammatory formulation, because it has been found to decrease multiple factors that contribute to joint inflammation. Indeed, many herbs possess anti-inflammatory powers. For instance, the active component of turmeric is curcumin, the yellow pigment of turmeric, a substance long used both topically and internally in Ayurvedic medicine, the indigenous system of medicine of India. Turmeric is a powerful antioxidant and anti-inflammatory, and effective in the treatment of sprains and inflammation.

In addition, curcumin offers antioxidant properties that prevent the formation and neutralization of existing free radicals—those terrorist, unstable, oxygen molecules that cause oxidation and premature aging in the body, setting us up for serious illnesses such as cancer and heart disease.

The curcumin in turmeric also stops precancerous changes within DNA and interferes with enzymes necessary for cancer progression. It also stops the oxidation of cholesterol, thus protecting against the formation of plaque in arteries.[94] In an experimental double-blind study, patients received either curcumin or phenylbutazone (300 mg per day). The improvements in the duration of morning stiffness, walking time, and joint swelling were comparable in both groups. However, while phenylbutazone is associated with significant adverse effects, curcumin has not been shown to produce any side effects at the recommended dosage level.[95]

– Green Tea Extract

Green tea possesses anti-inflammatory properties.[96] "One study showed that, when added to human cartilage cell cultures, the active ingredients in green tea inhibited chemical and enzymes that lead to cartilage damage and breakdown."[97] According to the National Center for Complementary and Alternative Medicine, laboratory tests suggests that green tea protects against cancer, improves mental alertness, and may possibly aid in weight loss, lower blood cholesterol, and protect the skin from sun damage. More studies need to be done.[98]

– Mixed Bioflavonoids

Bioflavonoids are essential for the proper absorption and metabolism of vitamin C. They assist vitamin C in keeping collagen, the intercellular cement, in healthy condition. That's why they are included in this anti-inflammatory formula. Bioflavonoids are vital because of their ability to increase the strength of the capillaries and regulate their permeability. These actions help prevent hemorrhages and ruptures in the capillaries and connective tissues and have been found to minimize bruising that occurs in contact sports.

– Bromelain and Papain

Bromelain is a mixture of enzymes found naturally in pineapples. Called a proteolytic enzyme because it helps in the digestion of proteins, it is one of the most popular supplements in Germany, according to the *Commission E Therapeutic Guide to Herbal Medicine,* which was developed by a special expert committee of the German Federal Institute for Drugs and Medical Devices. According to that guide, bromelain has been approved for the treatment of swelling, bruising, inflammation, and pain. It may help alleviate the pain of arthritis.[99]

Papain is another proteolytic enzyme. It is collected from unripe green papaya and used to enhance digestion. Papain has also been used to treat acute and chronic inflammations, poorly healing wounds, abscesses, and rheumatic and degenerative complaints.

– *Serratiopeptidase*

The body creates fibrin to protect an injured site from further harm. This tough fibrin can impede full healing and cause limited range of motion. Serratiopeptidase has a reputation for dissolving the fibrin formation by simply digesting it.

Serratiopeptidase has been used effectively to heal chronic inflammation in a number of ailments, especially chronic inflammatory ear, nose, or throat disorders. Although it has not been well studied in most medical fields, we have found it to be beneficial for our patients, and we have found two classic studies that support its reputation for offering powerful anti-inflammatory effects.

For example, in a classic multicenter, double-blind, placebo-controlled trial that investigated the clinical efficacy of the anti-inflammatory enzyme serrapeptase (a form of serratiopeptidase), Japanese researchers reported that oral cavity swelling had lessened in the serrapeptase-treated group.[100] Another multicenter, double-blind, placebo-controlled study, this one of 193 patients, revealed serrapeptase, "acts rapidly on localized inflammation" in ear, nose, and throat infections.[101]

– *Chymotrypsin*

The pancreas produces about 1.5 quarts of enzymatic secretions daily for the digestion and absorption of food. Chymotrypsin is one of these pancreatic enzymes. It is essential for proper protein digestion and useful in the treatment of many acute and chronic inflammatory conditions, including sports injuries, tendonitis, and rheumatoid arthritis.

– *Ginger Root*

Ginger fights inflammation, reducing spasms and cramps on a muscular level. Ginger is a strong antioxidant and effective antimicrobial agent for sores and wounds. In one study, eighteen patients with osteoarthritis took powdered ginger for periods ranging from three to thirty months. The journal *Medical*

Hypothesis reported that based on clinical observations, 100 percent of the patients who had reported muscular discomfort experienced relief in pain or swelling.[102]

In another study reported in the same article, twenty-eight patients with rheumatoid arthritis took powdered ginger for periods ranging from three to thirty months. Based on clinical observations, 75 percent of the patients reported relief from pain or swelling.[103]

In a third study, seven patients for whom conventional treatment had provided only temporary or palliative relief were treated with ginger. All reported substantial improvement, including pain relief, increased joint movement, and a decrease in swelling and morning stiffness.[104]

Studies like these were responsible for the addition of ginger root to our formulation.

– Omega 3

Research studies published almost daily report on the extraordinary benefits of omega 3 fatty acids from fish oils. A prime benefit often reported is relief from pain and inflammation. Apparently, omega 3 moderates the inflammatory response. The research studies also report that these fatty acids have protective effects against heart attack and stroke, promote better brain function, combat depression, and lower the risk of breast, colon, and prostate cancer. How could we not include them in this anti-inflammatory formulation?

Fish oil contains both docosahexaenoic acid (DHA) and eicosapentaenoic acid (EPA). "There is strong scientific evidence from human trials that Omega-3 fatty acids from fish or fish oil supplements (containing EPA+ DHA) significantly reduce blood triglyceride levels," according to information jointly provided by the US National Library of Medicine and the National Institutes of Health.[105] Furthermore, multiple randomized, controlled trials reveal patients reported improvement in morning stiffness and joint tenderness with regular intake of three to four grams of fish oil daily containing 700-900 mgs of the EPA component.

The Second Anti-Inflammation Formula

Our second anti-inflammatory formula is based on the enzymes pancreatin, bromelain, quercetin, Chinese skullcap, trypsin, serratiopeptidase, rutin, SOD, and chymotrypsin. We also included vitamin C and the minerals magnesium, manganese, and copper. We have already discussed those minerals and the synergistic effect set in motion when they are taken in conjunction with vitamin C. Now we look at the effectiveness of some of these additional key nutrients.

– Pancreatin (650 mg)

Our pancreas produces enzyme secretions that are required for the digestion and absorption of food. Enzymes secreted by the pancreas include lipase, which catalyzes (is the sparkplug behind) the breakdown of fats;[106] amylase, which is part of the action by which starch is broken down into simpler carbohydrates;[107] and protease, which catalyzes protein digestion and stimulates certain immune system cells.[108]

Pancreatic enzymes such as pancreatin are used to treat or prevent pancreatic insufficiency, which is characterized by impaired digestion, malabsorption, nutrient deficiencies, and abdominal discomfort. Physicians also prescribe pancreatic enzymes in the treatment of inflammatory and autoimmune diseases like rheumatoid arthritis, athletic injuries, tendonitis, cancer, and infections. Sometimes, our bodies just need a little extra help to do a great job.

Pancreatin supplementation can result in decreased food intake and a significant loss of body weight, because it appears to either contain or stimulate the manufacture of compounds that suppress appetite.[109]

– Bromelain (400 mg)

As mentioned previously, bromelain is the proteolytic enzyme of the pineapple. It can help reduce inflammation caused by rheumatoid arthritis and other ailments. The protease enzymes found in pineapple and papaya can aid in the destruction of hard bonds that form in the body during a process called cross-linking. Cross-linking is a process that results in such conditions as hard, inflexible arteries and wrinkled skin. At the molecular level, cross-linking causes the body to become stiff and less agile. Large molecules such as collagen, a protein in connective tissue, become welded together by those cross-links. These abnormal cells can cause aging as well as many other conditions, including cancer.[110]

Bromelain can prevent cross-linking and swelling after trauma. In one study involving 146 boxers, seventy-four received bromelain, and seventy-two did not. All signs of bruising were completely cleared within four days in fifty-eight of the seventy-four who received bromelain. Only ten of the boxers who did not take bromelain showed no signs of bruising at the end of the four days. The remainder took seven to fourteen days for their bruises to clear.

– Quercetin (300 mg)

Another substance that works well in combination with pancreatin and bromelain is quercetin. Combination preparations of protein-digesting enzymes such as these boost each other's anti-inflammatory activities.[111]

Quercetin is a powerful antioxidant and antihistamine found in the skins of red apples and red onions. It is also found in berries, tea, grapes, pineapples, and red wine. Research indicates that its anti-inflammatory properties can help reduce pain from arthritis and other inflammatory diseases. Its antihistamine actions can help relieve asthma and allergies. Quercetin may also help reduce symptoms like fatigue, depression, and anxiety.

– Rutin (100 mg)

Rutin, a bioflavonoid similar to quercetin, is listed in the *U.S. Pharmacopoeia* and identified as a potent anti-inflammatory. In fact, rutin and quercetin have been shown to work together to moderate inflammation. That's why both are added to many anti-inflammatory preparations. Rutin has also been shown to restore the antioxidant abilities of vitamin C after it neutralizes free radicals. Rutin also helps maintain collagen, the substance that keeps our skin healthy, elastic, and firm. It, along with quercetin, is considered useful in treating inflammatory diseases such as gout, arthritis, and inflammatory bowel disease.

– SOD (80 mg)

Superoxide dismutase (SOD) is an enzymatic antioxidant that removes the potentially toxic superoxide ion from the body by breaking it down into oxygen and hydrogen peroxide.[112] It acts as both an antioxidant and an anti-inflammatory in the body. In doing so, it helps protect the integrity of the joints and the immune system. It has been used to treat arthritis and other inflammatory diseases.

Conclusion

Our research and experience convince us that the formulations just discussed are safe and effective. They may prevent the development of conditions that could lead to surgery. However, it must be pointed out that this statement has not been evaluated by the FDA. That's because the FDA doesn't strictly regulate herbs or supplements. Consequently, there are no guarantees of strength, purity, or safety for any herbal product and their effects may vary.

You should always read product labels and know what you are putting into your body. If you have a medical condition or are taking other drugs, herbs, or supplements, you should speak with a qualified health-care provider before starting a new therapy. Consult a health-care provider immediately if you experience side effects or drug interactions.

Take-Home Points from Chapter 7

- Certain herbs and supplements may prevent the development of conditions that could lead to surgery.

- You should always read product labels and know what you are putting into your body.

- If you have a medical condition or are taking other drugs, herbs, or supplements, you should speak with a qualified health-care provider before starting a new therapy.

- Consult a health-care provider immediately if you experience side effects or drug interactions.

8

Other *Beyond the Knife* Therapies

Modern medicine and technology are advancing so fast that the treatment landscape is a whole new world compared to modalities of the early twentieth century. Many new treatments have been and continue to be developed to replace surgery for a wide variety of conditions, including cancers. Let's take a closer look at some of these therapies.

Hormone Replacement Therapy to Prevent Osteoporosis-Related Surgery

– Osteoporosis

Osteoporosis is a progressive, debilitating condition that, in its most severe form, causes fractures that are often treated with surgery. Ten million Americans have osteoporosis, while another thirty-four million have low bone mass, leaving them at increased risk for osteoporosis.[113]

Osteoporosis-related fractures usually occur in the hip, spine, or wrist. Not all fractures require surgery, but serious ones often do. For instance, if you experience a hip fracture due to osteoporosis, you may need surgery to repair your hip. In the US, 1.5 million osteoporotic fractures occur each year. Of those, seven hundred thousand occur in the spine.[114] Osteoporosis can also cause painful compression fractures and other back problems. Two surgical treatments, vertebroplasty and kyphoplasty, sometimes relieve that pain. Many people now take steps to avoid those surgeries.

Osteoporosis is a disease that destroys bone mass and makes bones more likely to break under stress. Most often afflicted are the bones of the spine, hips, and wrists. The National Osteoporosis Foundation estimates that approximately ten million Americans have osteoporosis, and another thirty-four million have low bone mass.[115]

Women are four times more likely to develop osteoporosis than men; eight million of the ten million Americans with osteoporosis are women. Women often lose up to 20 percent of their bone mass in the five to seven years following menopause. Lessened and weakened bone mass can cause painful spinal compression fractures.

Treatments to relieve pain from severe fractures and osteoporosis-caused spinal compression include vertebroplasty for spinal compression and kyphoplasty for fractures caused by osteoporosis-weakened bones. Those are the surgeries we try to avoid.

Research reveals that those operations may be avoided when estrogen replacement therapy (ERT) and hormone replacement therapy (HRT) are used as treatments.

Estrogen deficiency is one of the main causes of bone loss in women during and after menopause. ERT and HRT have been proven to reduce bone loss, increase bone density, and reduce the risk of hip and spinal fractures in postmenopausal women.[116]

There are two types of estrogens: bio-identical, which include estradiol, estrone, and estriol; and synthetic, such as Premarin and the "designer estrogens," including tamoxifen (Nolvadex) and raloxifene (Evista), which are selective receptor modulators (SERMs). There have been warnings that synthetic estrogens (including Premarin, which comes from equine [horse] urine) increase the risks of cancer. Indeed, the Women's Health Initiative study revealed in 2002 that hormone replacement pharmaceuticals, like Premarin (estrogen) and Prempro (estrogen and progestin) increase the risk of stroke and other serious problems, including breast cancer.

Nevertheless, the FDA maintains that synthetic hormone drugs designed to replenish female hormone levels lowered during menopause are safe. Here's a rundown on those drugs.

➤ Premarin

Premarin is composed of estrogenic compounds derived from the urine of pregnant mares. Introduced in 1949, it is viewed as the "gold standard" of the hormone replacement world.

Sales hit an all-time high during the 1980s and 1990s, when studies (many supported by Wyeth-Ayerst, the maker of Premarin) began to support estrogen's role in keeping the cardiovascular system healthy. For example, Premarin was shown to lower LDL cholesterol, which the famous Framingham study had identified as a risk factor for cardiovascular disease. In the 1980s and 1990s, Premarin seemed to do just about everything: lift depression, prevent heart disease, and even prevent osteoporosis.

Today, however, the use of HRT has become one of the most controversial topics in the area of women's health. Multiple studies have reported a link between supplementation with synthetic estrogen, including equine urine-based estrogen and breast cancer.

Does that risk outweigh the possible benefits of cardiovascular protection? Perhaps it does not.

At the turn of the twenty-first century, several large prospective studies challenged the cardiovascular protection assumptions of Premarin and other estrogens.[117]

Although some experts continue to believe that synthetic estrogen has a cardiovascular benefit, we can no longer assume that this is true for everyone.

➤ Bio-identical Hormones

Because of fear of the potential increased cancer risk, many women and their doctors turned to compounded bio-identical hormone replacement therapy (BHRT). BHRTs are synthesized in the lab from hormone precursors found in plants.

These custom-made drugs, available only with a licensed practitioner's prescription, consist of individualized doses of hormones, including estriol, that are claimed to be chemically identical to human hormones. Indeed, estriol is a weak estrogen some researchers believe provides some protection against breast and endometrial cancers.

However, the problem is that the risks of bio-identicals are undetermined. There are no long-term scientific studies proving that they work or that they are safe. The FDA issued a statement in 2007 that it was aware of no adequate randomized, prospective, controlled clinical trials of compounded BHRT drugs that either demonstrate they are better than a placebo at relieving menopausal symptoms or that compare them to an FDA-approved drug to establish that the compounded drugs work equally well. In fact, the FDA says it is a myth that bio-identical hormones are safer and more effective than FDA approved synthetic hormones.[118]

The actual FDA statement is as follows:

[The] FDA is unaware of any credible scientific evidence supporting the assertions that these bio-identical compounded products are a safe or effective alternative to FDA-approved drugs containing hormones.[119]

Bio-identical hormones, including estradiol, estrone, and estriol, cannot be patented, so pharmaceutical companies have no financial incentive to do expensive research and development in order to develop new products that contain them. This may account for the lack of expensive studies.

While the FDA recommends HRT, the FDA does not favor the use of bio-identical products. However, if you have tried Premarin or other equine urine–based products and the side effects have caused you to stop taking them, you may want to consider a bio-identically compounded product to protect your bones and replace the estrogen your body requires. Your doctor can give you a special prescription to take to a compounding pharmacy. Compounding services are now available even at Walgreens, a national chain.

Where Do We Go from Here to Protect Our Bones?

As the US population ages, the prevalence of osteoporosis will increase. The National Osteoporosis Foundation estimates that by 2020, 61 million men and women will have osteoporosis.[120] This number represents a lot of surgeries that may be avoided by proper preventive care!

To prevent osteoporosis in the first place, do the following:

- Avoid carbonated beverages. They leach calcium from your bones.

- Take calcium supplements to strengthen your bones.

- Exercise regularly to keep fit.

Some gravity or resistance type of exercise is essential. "Bones stay healthy only when they have vertical vectors of force placed on them regularly. A sedentary lifestyle provides insufficient weight-bearing exercise to stimulate bone growth," says Christaine Northrup, MD, author of the book, *The Wisdom of Menopause*. "Many studies have shown that bed rest is associated with osteoporosis. In contrast, weight training has been shown to build bone density even in post-menopausal women who aren't on estrogen."[121]

Keeping fit can help you avoid the risk of falling and fracturing bones, helping you avoid surgery. Here's a way of keeping fit and maintaining your balance that isn't written about much. I tell my patients of reports about a type of exercise known as gravity or inversion therapy, which appears to be useful in treating back problems caused by osteoporosis.

Another significant risk factor for osteoporosis is clinical depression. "Past or current depression in women is associated with decreased bone mineral density."[122] Talk to your doctor if you feel depressed. Exercise can also help you avoid clinical depression.

Most readers are already aware of the evidence of the adverse impact smoking and alcohol has on the health of our bodies. "Since smokers, along with women who consume two or more alcoholic drinks daily, are at highest risk for osteoporosis, women should refrain from smoking and limit alcohol intake.

Along with increased calcium, a second diet tip for maintaining strong bones is to reduce phosphate consumption. Phosphate consumption directly interferes with calcium absorption. Eliminate cola and root beer drinks, which are too high in phosphate.

A third tip is to limit caffeine. Caffeine increases the rate at which calcium is lost in the urine. Daily intake should be limited to no more than the equivalent of the caffeine in one or two cups of coffee.

Finally, be sure to include sources of boron in your diet. Boron is a trace element found in fruits, nuts, and vegetables. It has been found to reduce urinary calcium loss and to increase serum levels of 17-beta estradiol (the most biologically active estrogen); both of these effects help bone health. The minimum daily dose of boron needed (2 mg) per day is easily met with a diet rich in fruits, nuts, and vegetables; supplements can be taken up to 12 mg per day."[123]

Medicines to Combat Severe Osteoporosis

Besides HRT, other medicines have also been shown to combat osteoporosis and thus help women (and provide help to men for whom ERT and HRT are not appropriate) avoid surgery. Those medicines include alendronate sodium (Fosamax®), which is part of a group of medications called bisphosphonates. Bisphosphonates increase bone density and reduce the risk of fractures.

Other medicines that also reduce the rate of bone loss include:

- Risedronate sodium (Actonel®), which has similar effects as alendronate.

- Ibandronate sodium (Boniva®), a new type of bisphosphonate and taken only once a month. It works by slowing bone loss and may increase bone mass.

- If you have already been diagnosed with, or think you may be developing osteoporosis, see your doctor. Ask about the medical and nutritional supplement treatments (especially calcium supplements and bio-identical hormones) you can take to increase your health and well-being.

Keep in mind that weight-bearing exercise has been proven to increase bone density at any age. There is a type of exercise that is fun and suitable for you, whatever your physical condition. Even if you have back problems caused by osteoporosis, as mentioned earlier, you can participate in a gravity exercise known as inversion therapy. But, check with your doctor first.

Other Beyond the Knife
Alternatives to Surgery for Specific Conditions

– Extracorporeal Shock-Wave Lithotripsy for Kidney Stones and Heel Spurs

Kidney stones are one of the most excruciatingly painful conditions a person can suffer. Roughly one million Americans develop kidney stones each year. In the United States, approximately 10 to 15 percent of all adults will be diagnosed with a kidney stone in their lifetime.

During most of the twentieth century, the only way to remove the stones was through invasive surgery. Then, in the latter part of the 1980s, a machine known as the lithotripter was developed to do extracorporeal (outside the body) shock-wave (ESW) therapy.

Extracorporeal shock waves are high-energy acoustic waves generated by a process known as lithotripsy, in which high-frequency sound waves are transmitted through water and targeted at the afflicted area.[124] Since the waves only travel through water, the patient has to be seated in the bathtub-like extension of the lithotripter.

Extracorporeal shock (sound) waves are different from ultrasound, because they travel at a lower frequency and have no heating effect on the skin. The ESW waves travel through fluid and soft tissue until they strike an object with a different hardness, such as a bone or kidney stones. Properly targeted, the shock waves can demolish heel spurs and kidney stones. When they pass through the patient's body and hit the targeted site (kidney stones or heel spur), a tapping sensation may be felt as the stony material breaks up. It is generally painless.

The initial use of lithotripsy was to safely crush kidney stones in the body.[125] Later, the high-energy waves were used successfully to treat heel spurs (plantar fasciitis).[126]

– Plantar Fasciitis (Heel Spurs)

Plantar fasciitis is a common foot disorder that, before lithotripsy, was often resistant to non-operative treatment.

A randomized, placebo-controlled, multiply blinded crossover clinical trial that was reported in the *Journal of Bone and Joint Surgery* proved once and for all the effectiveness of ESW therapy for plantar fasciitis.[127] In this trial, following ankle-block anesthesia, each patient received one hundred graded shock waves. "For all 289 patients who had one or more actual shock wave treatment, 222 or 76.8 percent had a good or excellent result. No patient was made worse by the procedure." The researchers concluded, "electrohydraulic high-energy shock waves to the heel are a safe and effective noninvasive method to treat chronic plantar fasciitis."[128]

ESWs are certainly another example of an effective *Beyond the Knife* therapy.

– Better Chemotherapy for Colorectal and Other Cancers

Every year, approximately one hundred fifty thousand people are diagnosed with colorectal cancer. The standard therapy for colorectal cancer has been surgery followed by chemotherapy, but this may soon change. Now, there is a new study from a prestigious medical center that indicates multidrug chemotherapy can remove the need for surgery in most cases.

The study was done at New York's Memorial Sloan-Kettering Cancer Center. Principle investigator, Philip Paty, MD, who presented the findings at the American Society of Clinical Oncology's May 2009 annual meeting reported, "We've found that preemptive surgery to remove the primary tumor is almost always unnecessary."[129]

He said most colorectal cancer surgery is unnecessary. Because in most cases, the tumor won't grow larger and may, in fact, regress if state-of-the-art chemotherapy is used as the primary treatment instead of surgery. New chemotherapy drug regimes that shrink primary tumors, thus reducing the likelihood of potentially lethal complications, include 5-FU and leucovorin, irirotecan combined with 5-FU and leucovorin, and oxaliplatin plus capecitabine[130].

Dr. Paty and his fellow investigators reviewed the case histories of 233 patients treated for stage IV colorectal cancer at Sloan-Kettering from 2000 to 2006. All were treated with standard, state-of-the-art chemotherapy, sometimes combined with bevacizumab, an antibody that blocks the formation of blood vessels to tumors. According to the study, only sixteen patients developed problems that called for surgical intervention. The rest never required surgery.[131]

Naturally, each case of colorectal cancer is different. Some cases may need surgery before or after chemotherapy. If you have colorectal cancer and your doctor tells you surgery is the best treatment, ask him why. He may have a good reason, but if he says it is the standard therapy, you may be wise to question whether that is still true.

— Laser Therapy to Prevent Diabetic Amputations

Diabetes-associated circulatory and nerve damage is the leading cause of lower limb amputation in the United States, responsible for more than half of all foot and leg removals each year. According to the American Diabetes Association, 65,700 people lose a foot or a leg to diabetes every year.[132] Many people with diabetes are poor candidates for surgery because of complications from their disease, such as peripheral artery disease.

Conventional lasers were used briefly in the 1980s to burn away blockages within arteries. But, the technique was abandoned, because the heat from the laser was too damaging to surrounding healthy tissue. Now, a new laser technique that uses ultraviolet energy to restore blood flow to blocked arteries is helping people with advanced diabetes avoid amputation, one of the most devastating complications of diabetes.

The new laser is the xenon-hydrogen chloride excimer laser, which depends on flexible fiber optic catheters to deliver short bursts of ultraviolent energy to targeted sites on sick legs. The laser is able to target and vaporize blockages without damaging surrounding arteries. This feature reduces the potential of the formation of dangerous clots after the surgery.

In a peer-reviewed article published in the *Journal of Endovascular Therapy,* researchers described a study of 119 patients who were at high risk for amputation.[133] Fewer than one in ten (92 percent limb rescue rate) ended up having a foot or leg removed within six months after the use of the excimer laser.

"After nearly two decades of research and experimentation with laser-assisted angioplasty, the xenon-hydrogen chloride excimer laser emerged as the laser device best suited for the treatment of peripheral artery disease," writes the author of a 2009 review in a later issue of the same journal.[134]

Additional Nonsurgical Treatments

Besides laser therapy and chemotherapy, there are still other nonsurgical treatment options for various conditions.

Radiofrequency ablation involves the use of a special probe with tiny electrodes that kill cancer cells. Sometimes, the probe is inserted directly through the skin, and only local anesthetic is needed. In other cases, the probe is inserted through an incision in the abdomen. This is typically done in a hospital under general anesthesia.

Cryotherapy is a treatment that uses small, needle-like probes to freeze and destroy abnormal tissues, such as a group of cancer cells. Usually, only a tiny puncture through the skin is needed to insert the probes.

Let's learn more about these modalities.

— *Radiofrequency Ablation*

Radiofrequency ablation (RFA) is a minimally invasive nonsurgical procedure used not only for certain colorectal cases but also for liver and kidney tumors, back pain, varicose veins, and supraventricular tachyarrhythmia and other types of rapid heartbeats. A recent 2009 study, published in the *New England Journal of Medicine,* revealed that RFA is an effective treatment for dysplasia in people with Barrett's esophagus, a condition that can lead to deadly gastrointestinal cancer.[135] A related editorial in the journal called it a, "landmark study in the field."[136]

"Our results show there is a substantial difference between treatment with radiofrequency ablation and a placebo or sham treatment," said Nicholas Shaheen, MD, principal investigator of the study and an associate professor at the University of North Carolina (Chapel Hill) School of Medicine.[137]

➤ *Radiofrequency Ablation for Cancer*

RFA kills cancerous cells in the liver, kidneys, lungs, bones, and other organs by heating the cancerous cells and destroying them. The physician inserts a thin needle, guided by computed tomography (CT), through the skin and into the tumor. According to the Mayo Clinic, "the treatment is a less invasive alternative to surgery," used, "when surgery is not a good option for patients for various reasons, often when other medical conditions may increase the risk of surgery."[138] For instance, lung cancer patients with heart problems and/or poor pulmonary function may be candidates for RFA, especially if their cancerous tumors are limited in size and few in number.

RFA has been used to treat certain breast cancers, especially those that present in thousands of women with small, early tumors that have not spread to other areas of the body.

Dr. William Burak Jr., an oncologist at Ohio State University, says the procedure appears to be safe, relatively quick, and less invasive than a traditional lumpectomy. "We are pleased with the response. The women (patients) have all done well during the procedure," Burak said. "A lumpectomy, even though it is less problematic than a mastectomy, can still be disfiguring, and any time we can eliminate an invasive process, we help the patient."[139]

In most cases, a single tumor can be adequately treated in one session that usually takes less than one hour. The procedure is performed in the hospital, and the patient usually goes home the next day.

➤ *Back Pain and Radiofrequency Ablation*

Back pain is extremely common. Low back pain is the fifth most common reason for doctors' visits and accounts for more than $26 billion in direct health-care costs nationwide each year.[140] Surgery often fails to relieve back pain. Consequently, the trend in the United States is to avoid surgery for back pain. In fact, the American Pain Society in May 2009 issued new clinical practice guidelines for low back pain that emphasized using noninvasive treatments over invasive surgery.

RFA is a minimally invasive procedure that disables and prevents specific spinal nerves from transmitting pain signals. It is often recommended for patients with arthritis-related back or neck pain that has not responded to other treatments.

RFA may provide relief for months or even years. However, when the targeted nerves grow back, pain can—but does not always—return.

The procedure is administered while the patient is positioned face down on a padded X-ray table. The skin over the injection site is sterilized and numbed with a topical anesthetic. Doctors perform the entire procedure with fluoroscopic guidance. Fluoroscopy is a real-time X-ray device that allows the physician to see the patient's spine while guiding and positioning the radiofrequency transmitting needles.

Once the needles are positioned, the area (usually the sacroiliac joint) is again numbed and electrical signals are sent to the nerve endings, disabling the nerves' ability to transmit pain signals. Patients can usually expect significant reduction of their lower back pain within one to four weeks. The procedure is generally well tolerated with few minor complications, including swelling and bruising at the site of the treatment. These side effects go away after a few days.

➤ *Radiofrequency Ablation for Rapid Heartbeats*

Rapid heart rhythms account for a great majority of sudden cardiac deaths. According to the American Heart Association, RFA is a nonsurgical procedure used to treat some types of rapid heartbeat disorders, most often supraventricular tachyarrhythmias (rapid, uncoordinated heartbeats).[141] It is widely used, because it has a success rate of over 90 percent and a low risk of complications. It causes little or no discomfort, and patients can resume normal activities in a few days.

Again, a fluoroscope is used to guide the physician as he or she directs a catheter with an electrode at its tip to the area of the heart muscle that is the site of the rapid heartbeats. The fluoroscope helps the doctor place the catheter at the exact site inside the heart where radiofrequency energy (similar to microwave heat) is transmitted to the target cells that are transmitting the abnormal signals to the heart. The targeted cells in the nerve pathway are destroyed, so the extra impulses that caused the rapid heartbeats are blocked.

➤ *Radiofrequency Ablation for Varicose Veins*

Normally, blood circulates from the heart to the legs through arteries and back to the heart through veins that contain one-way valves that allow the blood to return from the legs against gravity. If these valves leak, blood pools in the veins of the leg, which become enlarged or varicose, meaning abnormally swollen and enlarged.

Varicose veins are a serious condition that usually progresses until surgery is needed, either by a "stripping" of the vein or by a procedure known as avulsion phlebotomy. RFA is used to seal off those faulty veins, diverting blood flow to nearby healthy veins. RFA has replaced certain types of vein stripping, because it is far less invasive than surgery and has lower complication rates. It is also, "well tolerated by patients and produces good cosmetic results," according to the Medscape Reference Drugs Conditions & Procedures website.[142]

— Cryotherapy

Cryotherapy is a minimally invasive treatment that uses extreme cold to freeze and destroy diseased tissue, including cancer cells. It is a commonly used procedure for the treatment of a variety of benign and malignant lesions, including prostate, liver, colorectal, and prostate cancers—especially when surgical resection is deemed to be too dangerous.

During cryotherapy, liquid nitrogen or argon gas is pumped through thin, needle-sized applicators called cytoprobes onto diseased cells located outside or inside the body. Radiologists use image-guidance ultrasound or computed tomography (CT scans), or magnetic resonance (MR) to guide the placement of the cytoprobes to treatment sites located inside the body.

Since cryotherapy is a percutaneous, image-guided procedure, it is most often performed by a specially trained interventional radiologist in a radiology suite, often on an outpatient basis. However, some procedures, such as prostate and liver cancer treatments, require hospital admission.

Typically, cryotherapy procedures are completed within one to three hours. At the end of the procedure, the cytoprobes are removed, and pressure is applied to stop any bleeding. The small opening in the skin is covered with a bandage. No sutures are needed.

➤ *Advantages of Cryotherapy*

Recovery time following cryosurgery for kidney or liver tumors is often less than when the tumor is surgically removed. Cryotherapy is less traumatic than surgery, since only a small puncture is needed to pass the probes through the skin. This limits damage to healthy tissue and causes less pain during and after the procedure. Consequently, overnight stays for pain relief are usually not needed.

Cryotherapy causes minimal scar tissue and no apparent calcifications. Indeed, fewer side effects are noted, compared to surgery. A patient can usually resume normal activities within twenty-four hours after the procedure. Patients are cautioned to avoid heavy lifting for several days if the cryotherapy was performed on or in the abdominal area.

Any interventional procedure also carries risks as well as benefits. Be sure to discuss your interest in these alternative treatments with your doctor, and always ask your doctor about the risks involved in any *Beyond the Knife* interventional procedures, including ESW therapy, RFA, or cryotherapy.

Take-Home Points from Chapter 8

- Estrogen deficiency is one of the main causes of bone loss in women during and after menopause. Bone loss sets up women for osteoporosis, which weakens bones and causes severe fractures and painful spinal compression that often require surgery. Estrogen replacement therapy (ERT) and hormone replacement therapy (HRT) can help many women avoid the necessity of surgery. ERT and HRT have been proven to reduce bone loss, increase bone density, and reduce the risk of hip and spinal fractures in postmenopausal women.[143]

- Laser therapy, extracorporeal shock wave therapy, radiofrequency ablation, and cryotherapy are *Beyond the Knife* alternatives to surgery for diseases and conditions ranging from prostate, liver, colorectal, kidney, and prostate cancers to gallstones, heel spurs, and varicose veins.

9

Beyond the Knife Future Therapies: Nanotechnology, Nanomedicine, and Gene Therapy

What if tiny robot doctors could search out and destroy the very first cancer cells that would otherwise have caused a tumor to develop in the body?

What if a broken part of a cell could be removed and replaced with a miniature biological machine?

What if pumps the size of molecules could be implanted to deliver life-saving medicines precisely when and where they are needed?

What if tiny robots—so tiny they would be invisible without the use of a microscope—were injected into the bloodstream and programmed to absorb, metabolize, or otherwise destroy and render harmless cancerous cells and other toxic substances, such as plaque blockages in the arteries?

These scenarios may sound like science fiction, but they are the long-term goals of the NIH's National Nanotechnology Initiative (NNI).[144] The NNI is a multi-agency US government program created in 2001 with the express purpose of, "accelerating the discovery, development, and deployment of nanometer-scale science."[145] The NNI coordinates the nanotechnology-related activities of twenty-six federal agencies, including the NIH.

The burgeoning field of nanotechnology creates myriad new opportunities for advancing medical science and in the treatment of disease. Scientists have long known that illness and disease are caused by damage on the molecular and cellular levels. Consequently, the NIH has invested over $8 billion in research since 2001 on nanotechnology and nanomedicine, and billions more on gene therapy research to investigate the molecular and cellular causes of diseases and illnesses.[146]

Nanotechnology, nanomedicine, and gene therapy all have mind-boggling potential. Unbelievable breakthroughs in all three fields are expected in the near future. Indeed, NIH scientists anticipate that research into these developing fields will yield astounding medical benefits as early as 2013.[147]

The term "nano" comes from the Greek word for "dwarf" and/or "extremely small." One nanometer (nm) is equal to one-billionth of a meter. To gain a sense of proportion, a double-strand of the DNA contained in a human cell has a diameter of 2 nm. The average cell is 1,000 nm. At the cellular level, a red blood cell is a "monster" at approximately 7,000 nm in diameter. In contrast, the diameter of a human hair is a mega-monster at approximately 80,000 nm.[148] The thickness of a single sheet of paper is 100,000 nm. So, picture this: 100 nm is equal to one hundredth of the thickness of the sheet of paper! (At its largest, nano materials are 100 nm. Above 100 nm, measurements change to a different scale of measurement.)

The conceptual foundation of nanotechnology research can be traced to Nobel Prize-winning physicist Richard P. Feynman, who spoke about the possibilities of manipulating materials at the scale of individual atoms and molecules in a prescient 1959 talk titled, "There's Plenty of Room at the Bottom." His talk was later published in the scientific journal *Engineering and Science.* According to that transcript, Feynman asked, "Why cannot we write the entire twenty-four volumes of the *Encyclopedia Britannica* on the head of a pin?"[149]

To accomplish that feat, he proposed the use of "machine tools to make smaller machine tools, those to be used to make still smaller machine tools, and so on all the way down to the atomic level."[150]

Nanomedicine is a subdivision of nanotechnology. Nanotechnology and nanomedicine are expected to make immense health benefits possible in drug delivery and in the monitoring, repair, construction, and control of human biological systems at the molecular level. For those things to occur, Feynman's "small machines" have to be built. Many are already on the drawing board, while some have already been built.

The term "nanotechnology" was born in 1974, when Norio Taniguchi, a researcher at the University of Tokyo, used it to describe the ability to engineer materials at the nanometer level.

Nevertheless, Feynman was the first scientist to suggest a medical use for "relatively small machines,"[151] which later were referred to as nanotechnology. Feynman, the "conceptual father" of nanotechnology, in his now-famous speech stated:

A friend of mine (Albert R. Hibbs) suggests a very interesting possibility for relatively small machines. He says that although it is a very wild idea, it would be interesting in surgery if you could swallow the surgeon. You put the mechanical surgeon inside the blood vessel and it goes into the heart. It finds out which valve is the faulty one and takes a little knife and slices it out. Other small machines might be permanently incorporated into the body to assist some inadequately functioning organ.[152]

Later, other scientists expanded the concept, speculating that millions of tiny nanorobots could be injected into the bloodstream to patrol the body to spot and cut out cancerous strands of DNA.

That's actually what will happen in the near future, according to R. A. Freitas, a nanotechnology textbook author and Senior Research Fellow of the Institute for Molecular Manufacturing in Palo Alto, California. He wrote:

It is always somewhat presumptuous to predict the future, but in this case we are on solid ground because most of the prerequisite historical processes are already in motion and all of them appear to be clearly pointing in the same direction.

The comprehensive knowledge of human molecular structure so painstakingly acquired during the twentieth and twenty-first centuries will be used in the twenty-first century to design medically-active microscopic machines. These machines, rather than being tasked primarily with voyages of pure discovery, will instead most often be sent on missions of cellular inspection, repair, and reconstruction. Nanomedicine will involve designing and building a vast proliferation of incredibly efficacious molecular devices, and then deploying these devices in patients to establish and maintain a continuous state of human healthiness.[153]

Indeed, there are various forms of nanotechnology already in use in nanomedicine. There are wound dressings that contain silver nanoparticles as a bactericide to kill germs,[154] stents coated with nanoporous drugs like hydroxyapatite that are used to keep arteries free of cholesterol and other lipids, as well as bone replacement materials, pacemakers, hearing aids that use nanomaterials, and sensors designed for the early detection of disease.

Nanotechnology Tools
Already Designed and in Existence

— *Nanoneedles*

With the aid of atomic force microscopy, nanoneedles have been fabricated from pyramidal silicon. A nanosurgeon could potentially perform an operation on a single cell without harming that cell.[155]

— *Nanotweezers*

Electrical voltages applied to nanoelectrodes are attached to carbon nanotubes, which open and close the free ends of those nanotubes, making, in effect, a nanotweezer. Researchers have already used a nanotweezer to manipulate submicron clusters. These devices could potentially be used by a nanosurgeon to move and manipulate specific organelles inside single cells.[156]

— *Nanosieves*

Among the earliest created therapeutically helpful nanomedical devices are nanosleeves.[157] In test laboratories, researchers have used micromachining techniques to manufacture tiny chambers within single crystalline silicon wafers in which biologic cells can be placed.[158] The chambers interact with the body's biologic environment through silicon filter membranes that have been micromachined to present a high density of uniform nanopores as small as 20 nm in diameter. The pores are large enough to allow small molecules—such as oxygen, glucose, and insulin—to pass but small enough to block the passage of toxic particles.

The first voltage-gated molecular nanosieve was fabricated at Colorado State University.[159] It had an array of cylindrical gold nanotubules with inside diameters as small as 1.6 nm. When those tubules were positively charged, the nanopores were "gated," and only negative ions could get through the nanotubules. That breakthrough has potential implications for nanodrug delivery (especially in diabetes) and for the creation of biologic nanosensors.[160]

Building on that work, diagnostic and therapeutic nanodevices can be created.

Starburst dendrimers are tree-shaped synthetic molecules up to a few nanometers in diameter. Dendrimers can be the single core of multi-component nano-sensing devices called tectodendrimers. A library of dendrimeric components could be synthesized to perform the following tasks:

1. Recognize diseased cells

2. Diagnose the disease state

3. Deliver the drug

4. Report location

5. Report therapy outcomes[161]

Experts point out that targeted delivery of superparamagnetic iron oxide nanoparticles (SPIONs) allow the accumulation of those iron oxide nanoparticles in metastatic cancer cells of peripheral tissues, lymph nodes, and bones. That accumulation will facilitate and enhance the sensitivity of MRI devices.[162] The experts say that SPIONs have already been tested in humans to discover breast cancer. They also say that future areas of nanoparticle research include pancreatic cancer.[163]

Future Applications of Nanotechnology and Nanomedicine

Cancer is the leading cause of death in the United States among individuals younger than eighty-five years of age. A horrible problem faced by cancer sufferers is that the chemotherapies given to kill the cancer cells in their bodies are also toxic to nontarget tissues. That's why people who are treated with chemotherapy often suffer from nausea and lose their hair. Nanotechnology-based delivery systems can prevent those potential side effects.

Perhaps the greatest immediate impact of nanotechnologies in cancer therapy will be in the realm of drug delivery. The best way to increase the efficacy and reduce the toxicity of a cancer drug is to direct the drug to its target and maintain its concentration at the site of the cancer long enough to allow therapeutic action to take effect. The therapeutic index of nearly all drugs currently being used would be improved if they were more efficiently delivered to their biological targets through the appropriate application of nanotechnologies.

Researchers at the University of Texas Health Science Center in San Antonio, the University of Texas Southwestern Medical Center in Dallas, and Baylor School of Medicine are already using nanotechnology to target, "micro metastases, tiny aggregates of cancer cells too small for surgeons to find and remove with a scalpel."[164] The three medical centers are involved in a pilot study involving human patients with head and neck cancer.

The *Beyond the Knife* therapy being used involves nanoshells containing gold-coated silica with different "optical resonances," depending on the size of its layers. These nanoshells, embedded in a drug-containing hydrogel polymer, are injected into the body near the tumor cells. When heated with an infrared laser, the nanoshells (each about the size of a polio virus) selectively absorb a specific infrared frequency, melting the polymer thus releasing the anti-cancer drug payload into the tumor.[165] A polio virus is only about 27–30 nanometers in diameter. To view it, a poliovirus has to be magnified some 450,000 times.[166]

The company producing the nanoshells is Nanospectra Biosciences, Inc., of Houston. Probably because of the gold-coated silica components of the nanoshell, the company calls its product AuroLase Therapy: "auro" is a prefix meaning gold or golden. Here's hoping the company's product helps those head and neck cancer patients. If it does, the rewards will certainly be golden.

— Fullerene Nanospheres also Show Great Promise

Another nanotechnology approach with that goal in mind is the development of Fullerene compounds. Fullerenes such as C_{60}, a soccer-ball-shaped arrangement of sixty carbon atoms per molecule, show great promise as pharmaceutical agents. These materials exhibit good biocompatibility and low toxicity, even at relatively high doses.

Nano-sized Fullerene balls have potential in the near future to serve as antiviral agents against HIV, for instance, and against bacterial agents such as Escherichia coli, streptococcus, and mycobacterium tuberculosis and as *Beyond the Knife* alternatives to surgery in anti-tumor and anticancer therapies. They may also be effective as treatments for amyotrophic lateral sclerosis and Parkinson's disease.[167]

A problem faced by pharmaceutical manufacturers is that certain drugs are not very chemically available in the body. Some, like Fullerene nanospheres, don't last long in the body, and that affects their usefulness. Novel nanotech drug delivery systems would offer protection to drugs which have short half-lives in the body.

— *Nanomedicine for Diabetes*

Soon, nanomaterials are also likely to help people with type 2 diabetes. One problem faced by people with type 2 diabetes is that the disease is progressive, and as diabetes progresses, their pancreas "burns out" and produces less and less insulin.

One of the simplest nanomedicine materials is a nanoshell, a surface perforated with nanopores. The pores are large enough to allow small molecules, such as glucose and insulin, to pass through. They are small enough, however, to interfere with the passage of much larger molecules, such as immunoglobulin and virus particles, that may attack the pancreas.

In one experiment, the pancreases of lab rats were protected by the nanoshell. Protected by the nanoshells, the rat pancreatic cells were allowed to receive nutrients and remain healthy for weeks. It is believed likely that what works on rats will work on humans. Studies are being readied to see if that experiment can be replicated.[168]

Freitas, the nanotechnology textbook author and Senior Research Fellow of the Institute for Molecular Manufacturing in Palo Alto, California, believes:

> Nanoshells might prove useful in treating diabetes—a patient would use a ballpoint-pen-sized infrared laser to heat the skin site where nanoshell polymer had been injected, releasing a pulse of insulin. Unlike injections, which are taken several times a day, the nanoshell-polymer system could remain in the body for months.[169]

Genetic Therapy and Nanotechnology Are Expected to Work Well Together

The operating systems of all living things—the networks of genes that make us who we are—are called genomes. The human genome has almost completely been mapped. At least a dozen cancer cell types have already been linked to at least one unique protein that targeting dendrimers could use to identify it as cancerous.

As the genomic and nonmedical revolutions progress, it is likely that proteins unique to every type of cancer will be identified, thus allowing the design of recognition dendrimers for each kind of cancer. Once recognized, those cancers can be targeted by nanodrug delivery systems specifically aimed at the cancer that needs to be cured. Although practical clinical (*Beyond the Knife*) therapies based on this knowledge are probably at least three to five years in the future, they are coming. Look for a cure for cancer and many other diseases. Nanotechnology and gene therapies will revolutionize medicine.

Gene therapy, the repair of malfunctioning cells by mending the DNA scripts that cause cells to function, offers a much-needed solution to diseases caused by a single flawed gene.

Unfortunately, since the first human gene therapy began in 1990, the field has struggled with technical challenges and setbacks, including the death of a volunteer in a clinical trial. Nevertheless, in 2009, gene therapy started galloping down the comeback trail as researchers reported success in treating several devastating diseases. Even more success is expected in the near future.

Diseases for which gene therapy is already successfully being used include Leber's congenital amaurosis (LCA), a rare form of inherited blindness that affects infants; X-linked adrenoleukodystropy (ADL), a destructive disease that too often killed boys before they became teenagers; and severe combined immunodeficiency (SCID; also known as the "bubble boy" disease), which makes children susceptible to early death from out-of-control infections.

The most common approach for correcting faulty genes is the insertion of a normal gene to replace a nonfunctional gene. (The nanotweezer might be helpful here.) However, present-day types of gene delivery systems—such as viral delivery and the direct injection of genetic material into the body—have potential problems. Those problems include concerns the virus involved in viral delivery may go "wild" and cause harm to the body, and there are worries about the immunogenicity of the viral vectors (whether the body can assimilate the viral vectors and not reject them).

Nanotechnology can ride to the rescue. Indeed, there is a race going on between scientific researchers to determine who will be the first to successfully designing safe and efficient gene delivery mechanisms using nanotechnology. As part of that race, researchers are trying to engineer bacterial "bio-robots." That's the source of the hope mentioned at the beginning of this chapter, "tiny robots—so tiny they would be invisible without the use of a microscope," will someday soon be, "injected into the bloodstream and programmed to absorb, metabolize, or otherwise destroy and render harmless cancerous cells and other toxic substances within the body such as plaque blockages in the arteries."

Textbook author Freitas believes, "In the longer term, perhaps 10 to 20 years from today [he was writing in 2005], the earliest molecular machine systems and nanorobots may join the medical armamentarium, finally giving physicians the most potent tools imaginable to conquer human disease, ill health, and aging."[170]

So, delivery of repaired genes and/or the destruction and replacement of incorrect genes are fields in which nanoscale treatment mechanisms are expected to be introduced successfully in the near future. The multidisciplinary fields of nanotechnology and genetic therapy are bringing the science of nanomedicine closer and closer to reality.

The effects of these developments will, at some point soon, be so vast they will probably affect virtually all medical specialties. Nanotechnology holds the promise of delivering the greatest medical breakthroughs in history. Over the next couple years, it is widely anticipated that nanotechnology, nanomedicine, and genetic therapy will continue to evolve and expand, resulting in many more *Beyond the Knife* treatment modalities. I can hardly wait.

Here's my ending message to you, dear reader: if you are scheduled for any type of surgery, google the various *Beyond the Knife* treatments described in this book, especially those described in this chapter, to find out if the future is already here for you. You may be able to avoid a scheduled surgery with *Beyond the Knife* therapies. Don't make any decisions, though, until you speak with a knowledgeable health-care provider. Surgery can be, and often is, a lifesaver. But, *Beyond the Knife* therapies already available or just beyond the horizon may do the job better. If they are still "beyond the horizon," however, and your physician says you need surgery now, don't delay! Act on the advice. Just know that someday we'll have a solution that is *Beyond the Knife*.

Take-Home Points from Chapter 9

- The term "nano" comes from the Greek word for "dwarf" and/or "extremely small." One nanometer (nm) is equal to one-billionth of a meter.[171]

- The burgeoning new field of nanotechnology creates myriad new opportunities for advancing medical science and in the treatment of disease. Scientists have long known that illness and disease are caused by damage at the molecular and cellular levels. Consequently, the NIH has invested over $8 billion in research since 2001 on nanotechnology and nanomedicine, and billions more on gene therapy research to investigate the molecular and cellular causes of diseases and illnesses.[172]

- Nanotechnology, nanomedicine, and gene therapy all have mind-boggling potential. Unbelievable breakthroughs in all three fields are expected in the near future. Indeed, NIH scientists anticipate that research into these developing fields will yield astounding medical benefits as early as 2013.[173]

Endnotes

Chapter 1

1. Baker S. Hospital-acquired superbug infections soar in newborn babies. Natural News website. 2010. http://www.naturalnews.com/026587_infections_superbug_health.html. Published July 9, 2009. Accessed April 1, 2011.

2. Johnson CK. Lax infection control at surgery centers. *Associated Press.* 2010. http://www.rdmag.com/News/FeedsAP/2010/06/life-sciences-study-lax-infection-control-at-surgery-centers. Published June 8, 2010. Accessed April 1, 2011.

3. Preidt R. The increased risk of staph infection of the brain [and] thoracic surgery. *HealthDay.* 2010. http://www.hanliumm1.com/the-increased-risk-staph-infection-of-the-brain-thoracic-surgery/. Published June 10, 2010. Accessed March 20, 2011.

4. Preidt R. The increased risk of staph infection of the brain [and] thoracic surgery. *HealthDay.* 2010. http://www.hanliumm1.com/the-increased-risk-staph-infection-of-the-brain-thoracic-surgery/. Published June 10, 2010. Accessed March 20, 2011.

5. Scott II DR; Division of Healthcare Quality Promotion, National Center for Preparedness, Detection, and Control of Infectious Diseases, Coordinating Center for Infectious

Diseases Centers for Disease Control and Prevention. The
direct medical cost of healthcare-associated infections in U.S.
hospitals and the benefits of prevention. 2009. **http://tinyurl.
com/6x4fyqo.** Published March, 2009. Accessed March 23,
2011.

6.   Klevens RM, Edwards JR, Richards CL, et al. Estimating
     health care-associated infections and deaths in U.S. hospitals,
     2002. *Public Health Reports.* 2007;122:160-166. http://www.
     cdc.gov/ncidod/dhqp/pdf/hicpac/infections_deaths.pdf. 2007.
     Published March-April, 2007. Accessed March 23, 2011.

7.   Workplace safety and health topics. mrsa and the workplace.
     Centers for Disease Control and Prevention website. http://
     www.cdc.gov/niosh/topics/mrsa/. Accessed April 1, 2011.

8.   Baker S. Hospital-acquired superbug infections soar in
     newborn babies. *Natural News.* 2009. http://www.naturalnews.
     com/026587_infections_superbug_health.html. Published July
     9, 2009. Accessed March 23, 2011.

9.   O'Reilly KB. MRSA surgical infections exact heavy clinical,
     financial toll. *amednews.* 2010. http://www.ama-assn.org/
     amednews/2010/01/11/prse0114.htm. Published January 14,
     2010. Accessed March 23, 2011.

10. Anderson DJ, Kaye KS, Chen LF, Schmader, KE, et al.
     Clinical and financial outcomes due to methicillin resistant
     staphylococcus aureus surgical site infection: a multi-center
     matched outcomes study. PLoS ONE website. 2009. http://
     www.plosone.org/article/info%3adoi%2f10.1371%2fjournal.
     pone.0008305#s1. Published December 15, 2009. Accessed
     March 23, 2011.

11. Anderson DJ, Kaye KS, Chen LF, Schmader, KE et al.
     Clinical and financial outcomes due to methicillin resistant
     staphylococcus aureus surgical site infection: A multi-center
     matched outcomes study. PLoS ONE website. 2009. http://
     www.plosone.org/article/info%3adoi%2f10.1371%2fjournal.
     pone.0008305#s1. Published December 15, 2009. Accessed
     March 23, 2011.

12. Gottrup F, Melling A, Hollander D A. An overview of surgical
     site infections: aetiology, incidence and risk factors. Key points.
     World Wide Wounds. 2005. http://www.worldwidewounds.

com/2005/september/Gottrup/Surgical-Site-Infections-Overview.html. Published September, 2005. Accessed March 23, 2011.

13. Institute for Healthcare Improvement. Surgical site infections: the case for improvement. http://www.ihi.org/IHI/Topics/PatientSafety/SurgicalSiteInfections. Accessed April 1, 2011.

14. Gottrup F, Melling A, Hollander D A. An overview of surgical site infections: aetiology, incidence and risk factors. Key points. *World Wide Wounds.* 2005. http://www.worldwidewounds.com/2005/september/Gottrup/Surgical-Site-Infections-Overview.html. Published September, 2005. Accessed March 23, 2011.

15. Yang H, Liang Ge, Hawkins BJ, Madesh M, et al. Inhalational anesthetics induce cell damage by disruption of intracellular calcium homeostatis with different potencies. *Anesthesiology: The Journal of the American Society of Anesthesiologists.* 2008;109(2):243-250.

16. IOS Press. Anesthesia increases risk of developing alzheimer's disease in patients with genetic predisposition. *Science Daily.* 2010 . http://www.sciencedaily.com/releases/2010/03/100324155359.htm. Published March 25, 2010. Accessed March 23, 2011.

Chapter 2

17. Hall S. *A Commotion in the Blood: Life, Death, and the Immune System.* New York: Henry Holt and Company; 1998:319.

18. Lee J. Identification of cell-specific soluble mediators and cellular targets during cell therapy for the treatment of heart failure. *Regenerative Medicine.* 2008;3(6):953–962.

19. Centers for Disease Control. February is American heart month: heart disease is the number one cause of death. http://www.cdc.gov/features/heartmonth/. Published January 31, 2011. Accessed March 23, 2011.

20. Pessina A, Grlbaldo L. The key role of adult stem cells: therapeutic perspectives. *Current Medical Research and Opinions.* 2006; 22(11):2288.

21. Pessina A, Grlbaldo L. The key role of adult stem cells: therapeutic perspectives. *Current Medical Research and Opinions.* 2006; 22(11):2293.

22. Tse HF, Kwong YL, Chan JKF, Lo G, Ho CL, Lau CP. Angiogenesis in ischaemic myocardium by intramyocardial autologous bone marrow mononuclear cell implantation. *Lancet.* 2003;361:47–49.

23. Tse HF, Kwong YL, Chan JKF, Lo G, Ho CL, Lau CP. Angiogenesis in ischaemic myocardium by intramyocardial autologous bone marrow mononuclear cell implantation. *Lancet.* 2003;361:47.

24. Pessina A, Grlbaldo L. The key role of adult stem cells: therapeutic perspectives. *Current Medical Research and Opinions.* 2006;22(11):2296.

25. Falanga V, Iwamoto S, Chartier M, Yufit T, Butmarc J, Kouttab N, Shrayer D, Carson P. Autologous bone marrow-derived cultured mesenchymal stem cells delivered in a fibrin spray accelerate healing in murine and human cutaneous wounds. *Tissue Engineering.* 2007;13:1299.

26. Marlovits S, Mousvi C, Gäbler J, Erdos J, Vécaei V. A new simplified technique for producing platelet-rich plasma: a short technical note. *European Spine Journal.* 2004;13 (Suppl 1):S102–S106.

27. Boyan BD. PRP in orthopaedics. AAOS Now website. 2010. http://www.aaos.org/news/aaosnow/sep10/cover2.asp. Published September, 2010. Assessed March 29, 2011.

28. Sampson S, Gerhardt M, Mandelbaum B. Platelet rich plasma injection grafts for musculoskeletal injuries: a review. *Current Review of Musculoskeletal Medicine.* 2008;1(3–4):165–174.

29. Doreal RJB, Sodre JCPP, Noronha, Cirurga Do Joelho, et al. Plasma rich growth factors and mesenquimal stem cells, a new strategy for treatment of knee chondral lesions: a case presentation. Paper presented at: 8th World Congress of the International Cartilage Repair Society; 2009; Miami, Fl. http://www.cartilage.org/index.php?pid=20. Accessed March 30, 2011; Filardo E, Kon M, Delcogliano A, Di Martino M, Lo Presti S, et al. PRP injections as treatment in chronic refractory jumper's knee: a controlled prospective study. Poster

presented at: 8th World Congress of the International Cartilage Repair Society; 2009; Miami, Fl. http://www.cartilage.org/index.php?pid=20. Accessed March 30, 2011.

30. Drapeau C. *The Stem Cell Theory of Renewal: Demystifying the Most Dramatic Scientific Breakthrough of Our Times.* Toronto, Ontario, Canada: Continental Shelf Publishing; 2008:28.

31. Drapeau C. *The Stem Cell Theory of Renewal: Demystifying the Most Dramatic Scientific Breakthrough of Our Times.* Toronto, Ontario, Canada: Continental Shelf Publishing; 2008:29.

32. Drapeau C. *The Stem Cell Theory of Renewal: Demystifying the Most Dramatic Scientific Breakthrough of Our Times.* Toronto, Ontario, Canada: Continental Shelf Publishing; 2008:29.

33. Drapeau C. *The Stem Cell Theory of Renewal: Demystifying the Most Dramatic Scientific Breakthrough of Our Times.* Toronto, Ontario, Canada: Continental Shelf Publishing; 2008:29–30.

34. Wrotniak M, Bielecki T, Gazdzik TSG. Current opinion about using the platelet-rich gel in orthopaedics and trauma surgery. *Ortopedia Traumatologia Rehabilitacja.* 2007;9(3):227–38.

35. Pessina A, Grlbaldo L. The key role of adult stem cells: therapeutic perspectives. *Current Medical Research and Opinions.* 2006;22(11):2288.

36. Choumerianous DM, Dimitriou H, Kalmanti M. Stem cells: promises versus limitations, *Tissue Engineering.* 2008;14(1, pt B):53–60.

37. Giordano GF, Rivers SL, Chung GK, Mammana RB, et al. Autologous platelet-rich plasma in cardiac surgery: effect on intraoperative and postoperative transfusion requirements. *The Annals of Thoracic Surgery.* 1988;46:416–419.

Chapter 3

38. Sampson S, Gerhardt M, Mandelbaum B. Platelet rich plasma injection grafts for musculoskeletal injuries: a review. *Current Review of Musculoskeletal Medicine.* 2008;3:165–174.

39. Angel M, Sgaglione N, Grande D. Clinical applications of bioactive factors in sports medicine: current concepts

and future trends. *Sports Medicine and Arthroscopy Review.* 2006;14(3): 38–145.

40. Creaney L, Hamilton B. Growth factor delivery methods in the management of sports injuries: the state of play. *British Journal of Sports Medicine.* 2008;42:314–320. http://dx.doi.org/10.1136/bjsm.2007.040071.

41. Sanchez M, Anitua E, Andia L. Use of a preparation rich in growth factors in the operative treatment of ruptured Achilles tendons. Poster Presentation at the 2nd International Conference on Regenerative Medicine. Miami, FL. 2005.

42. Elliott M. Tiger says he tore Achilles in 2008. AOL News website. 2010. http://www.aolnews.com/2010/04/05/tiger-says-he-tore-achilles-in-2008/. Published April 10, 2010. Accessed April 1, 2011.

43. Creaney L, Hamilton B. Growth factor delivery methods in the management of sports injuries: the state of play. *British Journal Sports Medicine,* 42:314–320. Published online November 5, 2007. http://dx.doi.org/10.1136/bjsm.2007.040071.

44. Wrotniak M, Bielecki T, Gazdzik T. Current opinion about using platelet-rich gel in orthopaedics and trauma surgery. *Ortopedia Traumatologia Rehabilitacja.* 2007;9(3):235.

Chapter 4

45. Handout on health: osteoarthritis. National Institute of Arthritis and Musculoskeletal and Skin Diseases website. http://www.niams.nih.gov/Health_Info/Osteoarthritis/#2. Published July, 2010. Accessed April 1, 2011.

46. Focht B, Rejeski W, Ambrosius W, Katula J, Messier S. Exercise, self-efficacy, and mobility performance in overweight and obese older adults with knee osteoarthritis. *Arthritis and Rheumatism.* 2005;53:659–665.

47. Ibrahirn V, Green B. Platelet Rich Plasma: an emerging treatment in sports medicine. National Rehabilitation Hospital website. 2011. http://www.nrhrehab.org/About+NRH/News+Archive/1098.aspx. Published 2011. Accessed April 1, 2011.

48. Arthritis Foundation. Osteoarthritis fact sheet. *News from the Arthritis Foundation.* Arthritis Foundation website. 2008. http://www.arthritis.org/media/newsroom/media-kits/Osteoarthritis_fact_sheet.pdf. Published 2008. Accessed April 1, 2011.

49. Comer AM, McGuire S. The pharma report: top 20 pharma companies. *Medical Marketing & Media.* 2008;45–55.

50. Kojima M, Kojima T, Suzuki S, Oguchi T, et al. Depression, inflammation, and pain in patients with rheumatoid arthritis. *Arthritis Care & Research.* 2009;61(8): 1018–1024.

51. Dean D. Nightshade vegetables may cause adverse reactions. *Natural News.* 2010. http://www.naturalnews.com/027978_nightshade_vegetables.html. Published January 20, 2010. Accessed March 23, 2011.

52. Chen F, Tuan R. Mesenchymal stem cells in arthritic diseases. *Arthritis Research and Therapy.* 2008;10(5):223.

Chapter 5

53. Mishra A, Woodall J Jr, Vieira A. Treatment of tendon and muscle using platelet rich plasma, *Clinics in Sports Medicine.* 2009;28(1):113–125.

54. Initially, the PRP procedure may cause some localized soreness and discomfort. Most patients only require some Extra-Strength Tylenol to help with the pain. Ice and heat can also be applied to the treated area as needed. After the injection of PRP, there can be increasing discomfort for approximately one to two weeks. Healing isn't instantaneous. While response times vary, the positive effects of the injection often take about six weeks to maximize. We recommend normal activity with no extra exercise for the first forty-eight hours. After ten to twelve days, patients can start light exercise. Heavy, stressful exercise before six weeks could result in incomplete healing of the treated tissue.

Chapter 5

55. Mishra A, Pavelko T. Treatment of chronic elbow tendinosis with buffered platelet rich plasma. *The American Journal of Sports Medicine.* 2006;34(11):1774–1778.

56. Mishra A, Pavelko T. Treatment of chronic elbow tendinosis with buffered platelet rich plasma. *The American Journal of Sports Medicine.* 2006;34(11):1774–1778.

Chapter 6

57. Barnes PM, Bloom B, Nahin RL. Complementary and alternative medicine use among adults and children: United States, 2007. *National Health Statistics Reports.* 2008; 12:1.

58. National Center for Complementary and Alternative Medicine. Americans spent $33.9 billion out-of-pocket on complementary and alternative medicine. *Disease Prevention Week.* 2009;2009:163.

59. Breecher MM. Complementary and alternative therapies frequently used by spine patients. *Doctor's Guide.* 2003. http://www.docguide.com/news/content.nsf/news/8525697700573E1 885256DD40050834. Published November 4, 2003. Accessed March 23, 2011.

60. Barnes PM, Bloom B. Complementary and Alternative Medicine Use Among Adults and Children: United States, 2007. 2008. http://tinyurl.com/4hc4a2b/. Published December 10, 2008. Accessed March 24, 2011.

61. Munshi A, Lee Hsueh NI, Tiwana MS. Complementary and alternative medicine in present day oncology care: promises and pitfalls. *Japanese Journal of Clinical Oncology.* 2008;38(8):512–520.

62. Tan K, Liu C, Chen A, Ding Y, Jin H, Seow-Choen F. The role of traditional Chinese medicine in colorectal cancer treatment. *Tech Coloproctol.* 2008;(12):1–6.

63. Wong R, Sagar C, Sagar S. Integration of Chinese medicine into supportive cancer care: a modern role for an ancient tradition. *Cancer Treatment Reviews.* 2001;(27):245–246.

64. Chopra A, Doiphode VV. Ayurvedic medicine: core concept, therapeutic principles, and current relevance. *Med Clinics of North America.* 2002;86:75–89.

65. Arnault I, Auger J. Seleno-compounds in garlic and onion. *Journal Chromatoge.* 2006; (1112):23–30.

66. Arnault I, Auger J. Seleno-compounds in garlic and onion. *Journal Chromatoge.* 2006; (1112):23–30.

67. Saper RB, Kales SN, Paquin J. Heavy metal content of Ayurvedic herbal medicine products. *Journal of the American Medical Association.* 2004;(292):2868–2873.

68. Tan K, Liu C, Chen A, Ding Y, Jin H, Seow-Choen F. The role of traditional Chinese medicine in colorectal cancer treatment. *Tech Coloproctol.* 2008;(12):1–6.

69. Tan K, Liu C, Chen A, Ding Y, Jin H, Seow-Choen F. The role of traditional Chinese medicine in colorectal cancer treatment. *Tech Coloproctol.* 2008;(12):5.

70. Tan K, Liu C, Chen A, Ding Y, Jin H, Seow-Choen F. The role of traditional Chinese medicine in colorectal cancer treatment. *Tech Coloproctol.* 2008;(12):5.

71. Tan K, Liu C, Chen A, Ding Y, Jin H, Seow-Choen F. The role of traditional Chinese medicine in colorectal cancer treatment. *Tech Coloproctol.* 2008;(12):2.

72. Thie J. *Touch for Health.* Revised Edition 2005. Los Angeles: DeVorss & Company; 2005:17.

73. Jacobson J, Workman S, Kronenberg F. Research on complementary/alternative medicine for patients with breast cancer: a review of the biomedical literature. *Journal of Clinical Oncology.* 2000;(18):668–683.

74. Dibble SL, Chapman J, Mack KA, Shih AS. Acupressure for nausea: results of a pilot study. *Oncology Nursing Forum.* 2000;27:41–47.

75. Manni L, Albanesi M, Guaragn M, Barbaro PS, Aloe L. Neurotropins and acupuncture. *Autonomic Neuroscience: Basic & Clinical.* 2010;157(1-2):9-17. Autonomic Neuroscience website. http://www.autonomicneuroscience.com/article/ S1566-0702%2810%2900067-6/. Published October 28, 2010. Accessed March 24, 2011.

76. Tjoa C, Pare E, Kim DR. Unipolar depression during pregnancy: non pharmacologic treatment options. *Women's Health.* 2010;6(4):565–576.

77. Mustian KM, Katula JA, Gill DL, Roscoe JA, Lang D, Murphy K, et al. Health-related quality of life and self-esteem: a randomized trial with breast cancer survivors. *Supportive Care in Cancer.* 2004;12:871–876.

78. Olson K, Hanson J, Michaud M. A phase II trial of Reiki for the management of pain in advanced cancer patients. *Journal of Pain Symptom Management.* 2003;(26):900–907.

79. Olson K, Hanson J, Michaud M. A phase II trial of Reiki for the management of pain in advanced cancer patients. *Journal of Pain Symptom Management.* 2003;26:900–907.

80. Munshi A, Lee Hsueh NI, Tiwana MS. Complementary and alternative medicine in present day oncology care: Promises and pitfalls. *Japanese Journal of Clinical Oncology.* 2008;38(8):519.

Chapter 7

81. Singh G. Recent considerations in non-steroidal anti-inflammatory drug gastropathy. *American Journal of Medicine.* 1998;105(1B):31S–38S.

82. Block G, Jensen CD, Norkus EP, Dalvi TB, Wong LG, McManus JF, Huddes, ML. Usage patterns, health, and nutritional status of long-term multiple dietary supplement users: a cross-sectional study. *Nutrition Journal.* 2007;6(30):6-30. Nutrition Journal website. http://www.nutritionj.com/content/6/1/30. Published October 24, 2007. Accessed March 23, 2011.

83. Dickinson A, Boyon N, Shao A. Physicians and nurses use and recommend dietary supplements: report of a survey. *Nutrition Journal.* 2009;1(8):29.

84. Das DK, Maulik N. Resveratrol in cardioprotection: a therapeutic promise of alternative medicine. *Molecular Interventions.* 2006;6(1):36.

85. Renaud S, de Lorgeril M. Wine, alcohol, platelets, and the French paradox for coronary heart disease. *Lancet.* 1992;339:1523–1526.

86. Harikumar KB, Aggarwal BB. Resveratrol: A multi-targeted agent for age-associated diseases. *Cell Cycle.* 2008;7(8):1020–1035. http://www.landesbioscience.com/journals/cc/article/5740. Published April 15, 2008. Accessed March 24, 2011.

87. Sawitzke AD, Clegg DO, Shi H, Finco MF, Dunlop DD, et al. The effect of glucosamine and/or chondroitin sulfate on the progression of knee osteoarthritis: a report from the glucosamine/chondroitin arthritis intervention trial. *Arthritis Rheumatism.* 2008;60(11):3314–3315.

88. Clegg DO, Reda DJ, Harris CL, Klein MA, O'Dell JR, Hooper MM, Bradley JD. Glucosamine, chondroitin sulfate, and the two in combination for painful knee osteoarthritis. *New England Journal of Medicine.* 2006;354(8):795–808.

89. Balch P, Balch J. *Prescription for Nutritional Healing.* New York: Avery Books; 2002:72.

90. Sawitzke AD, Shi H, Finco MF, Dunlop DD, Harris CL, Singer NG, et al. Clinical efficacy and safety of glucosamine, chondroitin sulphate, their combination, celecoxib or placebo taken to treat osteoarthritis of the knee: 2-year results from GAIT. *Annuals of Rheumatism Disease.* 2010;69(8): 1459–64. http://ard.bmj.com/content/69/8/1459.long. Published August, 2010. Accessed March 23, 2011.

91. Rothenberg M, Chapman C. *Dictionary of Medical Terms.* Hauppauge, NY: Barron's Educational Series; 2002:267.

92. Blain EJ, Ahmed Y, Ali VC. *Boswellia frereana* (frankincense) suppresses cytokine-induced matrix metalloproteinase expression and production of pro-inflammatory molecules in articular cartilage. *Journal of Phytotherapy Research.* 2009;24(6):905.

93. Blain EJ, Ahmed Y, Ali VC. *Boswellia frereana* (frankincense) suppresses cytokine-induced matrix metalloproteinase expression and production of pro-inflammatory molecules in articular cartilage. *Journal of Phytotherapy Research.* 2009;24(6):906.

94. Balch P, Balch J. *Prescription for Nutritional Healing.* New York: Avery Books; 2002:55.

95. Deodhar SD, et al. Preliminary studies on antirheumatic activity of curcumin (diferuloyl methane). *Ind J Med Res.* 1980;71: 632–634.

96. Handout on health: osteoarthritis. National Institute of Arthritis and Musculoskeletal and Skin Diseases website. http://www.niams.nih.gov/Health_Info/Osteoarthritis/. Published July 2010. Accessed March 24, 2011.

97. Handout on health: osteoarthritis. National Institute of Arthritis and Musculoskeletal and Skin Diseases website. http://www.niams.nih.gov/Health_Info/Osteoarthritis/. Published July 2010. Accessed March 24, 2011.

98. National Center for Complementary and Alternative Medicine. Green tea: what the science says. National Institutes of Health; Complementary and Alternative Medicine website. http://nccam.nih.gov/health/greentea/#science. Published May, 2006. Updated July, 2010. Accessed March 29, 2011.

99. Blumenthal M, Busse WR, Goldberg A, Gruenwald J, Hall T, Riggins CW, Rister RS. *The Complete German Commission E Monographs: Therapeutic Guide to Herbal Medicines.* Austin, TX: The American Botanical Council; 1998:94.

100. Tachibana M, Mizukoshi O, Harada Y, Kawamoto K, Nakai Y. A multi-centre, double-blind study of serrapeptase versus placebo in post-antrotomy buccal swelling. *Pharmatherapeutica.* 1984;3(8):526–530.

101. Mazzone A, Catalani M, Costanzo M, Drusian A, Mandoli A, Russo S, Guarini E, Vesperini G. Evaluation of serratia peptidase in acute or chronic inflammation of otorhinolaryngology pathology. *Journal of International Medical Research.* 1990;18(5):379–388.

102. Srivastava K, Mustafa T. Ginger in rheumatism and musculoskeletal disorders. *Med Hypothesis.* 1992;39:342–343.

103. Srivastava K, Mustafa T. Ginger in rheumatism and musculoskeletal disorders. *Med Hypothesis.* 1992;39:344–345.

104. Srivastava K, Mustafa T. Ginger in rheumatism and musculoskeletal disorders. *Med Hypothesis.* 1992;39:346–348.

105. National Institutes of Health. Fish Oil. Medline Plus Website. http://www.nlm.nih.gov/medlineplus/druginfo/natural/patient-fishoil.html. Published July 2010. Accessed April 1, 2011.

106. Rothenberg M, Chapman C. *Dictionary of Medical Terms.* Hauppauge, NY: Barron's Educational Series; 2002:232.

107. Rothenberg M, Chapman C. *Dictionary of Medical Terms.* Hauppauge, NY: Barron's Educational Series; 2002:29.

108. Kirschmann J, Dunne L. *Nutrition Almanac.* Columbus, OH: McGraw-Hill Book Company; 1984:213.

109. Murray M. *Encyclopedia of Nutritional Supplements.* Roseville, CA: Prima Publishing; 1996:398.

110. Kirschmann J, Dunne L. *Nutrition Almanac.* Columbus, OH: McGraw-Hill Book Company; 1984:213.

111. La Vecchia C, Negri E, Franceschi S, D'Avanzo B, Boyle P. Tea consumption and cancer risk. *Nutr Cancer.* 1992;17:27–31.

112. Valdiva A, Pèrez-Alvarez S, Aroca-Aguilar JD, Ikuta I, Jordán J. Superoxide dismutases: a physiopharmacological update. *Journal of Physiological Biochemistry.* 2009;65(2):195–208.

Chapter 8

113. Lin J, Lane JM. Osteoporosis. Medscape Reference Drugs Conditions & Procedures website. http://emedicine.medscape.com/article/1267595-overview. Updated April 30, 2009. Accessed April 1, 2011.

114. Lin J, Lane JM. Osteoporosis. Medscape Reference Drugs Conditions & Procedures website. http://emedicine.medscape.com/article/1267595-overview. Updated April 30, 2009. Accessed April 1, 2011.

Chapter 9

115. University of Virginia Health System. What is osteoporosis? http://www.healthsystem.virginia.edu/UVaHealth/adult_orthopaedics/osteopor.cfm. Published 2007. Accessed December 11, 2009.

116. Prince RL, Smith M, Dick IM, Price RI, et al. Prevention of postmenopausal osteoporosis: a comparative study. *Obstetrical & Gynecological Survey.* 1992;47(3):208–211.

117. Contreras I, Parra D. Estrogen replacement therapy: heart and estrogen/progestin replacement study. *American Journal of Health System Pharmacy.* 2000;57(21). Medscape Today News website. http://www.medscape.com/viewarticle/406921_5. Published February 15, 2010. Accessed April 1, 2011.

118. Food and Drug Administration. Bio-identicals: Sorting myths from facts. FDA Consumer Updates. US Food and Drug Administration website. http://www.fda.gov/ForConsumers/ConsumerUpdates/ucm049311.htm. Updated March 20, 2011. Accessed April 1, 2011.

119. Galson SK. Statement on pharmacy compounding/compounding of bio-identical hormone replace therapies for the Center for Drug Evaluation and Research Food and Drug Administration before the Senate Special Committee on Aging; April 19, 2007. US food and Drug Administration website. http://www.fda.gov/NewsEvents/Testimony/ucm154031.htm. Updated July 6, 2009. Accessed April 1, 2011.

120. Fisher J. Osteoporosis…it matters. National Osteoporosis Foundation website. http://www.nof.org/search/node/Osteoporosis%20in%202020. Published May 1, 2006. Updated September 24, 2010. Accessed April 1, 2011.

121. Northrup, C. *The Wisdom of Menopause.* New York: Bantam Books; 2001:378.

122. Michaelson D, Stratakis C, Hill L, et al. Bone mineral density in women with depression. *New England Journal of Medicine.* 1996;(335):1176–1181.

123. Northrup C. *Women's Bodies, Women's Wisdom.* New York: Bantam books; 1998:552–554.

124. Rompe JD, Decking J, Schoellner C, Nafe B. Shock wave application for chronic plantar fasciitis in running athletes: a prospective, randomized, placebo-controlled trial. *The American Journal of Sports Medicine.* 2009;31(2):268–274.

125. Sheir KZ, Madbouly K, Elsobky E, Abdelkhalek M. Extracorporeal shock wave lithotripsy in anomalous kidneys:

11-year experience with two second-generation lithotripters. *Urology*. 2003;(62):10–16.

126. Li X, Mengshi C, Lei L, Hai Q, Zhimin Z. Extracorporeal shock wave therapy: A potential adjuvant treatment for peri-implantitis. *Medical Hypotheses*. 2010. http://dx.doi. org/10.1016/j.mehy.2009.07.025. Published August 10, 2009. Accessed March 29, 2011.

127. Ogden JA, Alvarez RG, Levitt RL, et al. Electrohydraulic high-energy shock-wave treatment for chronic Plantar Fasciitis. *The Journal of Bone and Joint Surgery*. 2004;86:2216.

128. Ogden JA, Alvarez RG, Levitt RL, et al. Electrohydraulic high-energy shock-wave treatment for chronic Plantar Fasciitis. *The Journal of Bone and Joint Surgery*. 2004;86:2220.

129. Paty P. Metastatic colorectal cancer: Is Surgery Necessary? *Journal of the National Cancer Institute*. 2009;101(16):1113.

130. Paty P. Metastatic colorectal cancer: Is Surgery Necessary? *Journal of the National Cancer Institute*. 2009;101(16):1114.

131. Paty P. Metastatic colorectal cancer: Is Surgery Necessary? *Journal of the National Cancer Institute*. 2009;101(16):1115.

132. American Diabetes Association. Diabetes Statistics. Diabetes Basics. American Diabetes Association website. http:// www.diabetes.org/diabetes-basics/diabetes-statistics/?utm_ source=WWW&utm_medium=DropDownDB&utm_ content=Statistics&utm_campaign=CON. Released January 26, 2011. Accessed April 1, 2011.

133. Laird JR, Zeller T, Gray BH, Scheinert D, Vranic M, Reiser C, Biamino G. Limb salvage following laser-assisted angioplasty for critical limb ischemia: results of the LACI multicenter trial. *J Endovasc Ther*. 2006;13(1):1–11.

134. Das TS. Excimer laser-assisted angioplasty for infrainguinal artery disease. *Journal of Endovascular Surgery*. 2009;15(Suppl 2):1198.

135. Shaheen N. Radiofrequency ablation in barrett's esophagus with dysplasia. *New England Journal of Medicine*. 2009;360(22): 2277.

136. Shaheen N. Radiofrequency ablation in barrett's esophagus with dysplasia. *New England Journal of Medicine.* 2009;360(22):2278.

137. Shaheen N. Radiofrequency ablation in barrett's esophagus with dysplasia. *New England Journal of Medicine.* 2009;360(22):2277–2284.

138. Mayo Clinic. Radiofrequency ablation for cancer. Mayo Clinic website. http://www.mayoclinic.org/radiofrequency-ablation. Accessed March 25, 2011.

139. Burak W Jr. New treatment may eliminate need for surgery. http://tinyurl.com/2cxnvc2. Published May, 2002. Accessed March 29, 2011.

140. Oregon Health & Science University. New guideline for low-back pain interventions, surgery. *ScienceDaily.* http://www.sciencedaily.com/releases/2009/05/090513173457.htm. Published May 18, 2009. Accessed March 30, 2011.

141. American Heart Association. Radiofrequency ablation. American Heart Association website. http://www.heart.org/HEARTORG/Conditions/Arrhythmia/PreventionTreatmentofArrhythmia/Ablation_UCM_301991_Article.jsp. Updated July 21, 2010. Accessed March 23, 2011.

142. Weiss R, Feied CF, Weiss M. Varicose veins treated with radiofrequency ablation therapy. Medscape Reference Drugs Conditions & Procedures website. 2009. http://emedicine.medscape.com/article/1085800-overview. Updated September 2, 2009. Accessed March 29, 2011.

143. Prince RL, Smith M, Dick IM, Price RI, et al. Prevention of postmenopausal osteoporosis: a comparative study. *Obstetrical & Gynecological Survey.* 1992;47(3):208–211.

144. NIH Common Fund. *Nanomedicine Overview.* 2010. National Institutes of Health Website. http://nihroadmap.nih.gov/nanomedicine/index.asp. Published 2010. Accessed March 25, 2011.

145. The National Nanotechnology Initiative. Research and development leading to a revolution in technology and Industry: Supplement to the President's FY 2008 Budget. Washington, DC: The US Government; 2007:3.

146. The National Nanotechnology Initiative. Research and development leading to a revolution in technology and Industry: Supplement to the President's FY 2008 Budget. Washington, DC: The US Government; 2007:6.

147. Freitas RA Jr. What is Nanomedicine? *Nanomedicine: Nanotechnology, Biology, and Medicine.* 2005;1(1):325.

148. Sahoo SK, Parveen S, Panda JJ. The present and future of nanotechnology in human health care. *Nanomedicine: Nanotechnology, Biology, and Medicine.* 2007;3(1):20–31.

149. Feynman RP. There's plenty of room at the bottom. *Engineering and Science.* 1960; 23:22–36. http://www.zyvex.com/nanotech/feynman.html. Published 2006. Accessed March 25, 2011.

150. Asiyanbola B, Soboyejo W. For the surgeon: an introduction to nanotechnology. *Journal of Surgical Education.* 2008;65(2):155.

151. Feynman RP. There's plenty of room at the bottom. *Engineering and Science.* 1960; 23:22–36. http://www.zyvex.com/nanotech/feynman.html. Published 2006. Accessed March 25, 2011.

152. Feynman RP. There's plenty of room at the bottom. *Engineering and Science.* 1960; 23:22–36. http://www.zyvex.com/nanotech/feynman.html. Published 2006. Accessed March 25, 2011.

153. Freitas RA Jr. *Nanomedicine: Basic Capabilities* I. Georgetown, TX: Landes Bioscience; 1999:3–9.

154. Tian J, Wong KK, Ho CM, et al. Topical delivery of silver nanoparticles promotes wound healing. *Chem Med Chem.* 2006;2(1):129–136.

155. Han SW, Nakamura C, Obataya I, Nakamura N, Miyake J. A molecular delivery system by using AFM and nanoneedle. *Biosensors and Bioelectronics.* 2005;20(15):2120–2125.

156. Kim P, Lieber CM. Nanotube nanotweezers. *Science.* 1999;286(5447):2148–2150.

157. Desai TA, Chu TJK, Beattie JM, Hayek A, Ferrari M. Microfabricated immunoisolating biocapsules. *Biotechnology, Bioengineering.* 1998;57(1):118–120.

158. Lee SB, Martin CR. Electromodulated molecular transport in gold-nanotube membranes. *Journal of the American Chemical Society.* 2002;124(40):11850–11851.

159. Nishizawa M, Menon VP, Martin CR. Metal nanotube membranes with electrochemically switchable ion-transport selectivity. *Science.* 1995;68(3):700–702.

160. Leoni L, Desai TA. Micromachined biocapsules for cell-based sensing and delivery. *Advanced Drug Delivery Research.* 2004; 56(2):228.

161. Quintana A, Raczka E, Pichler L, et al. Design and function of a dendrimer-based therapeutic nanodevice targeted to tumor cells through the folate receptor. *Pharmaceutical Research.* 2002;19(9):1310–1316.

162. Asiyanbola B, Soboyejo W. For the surgeon: an introduction to nanotechnology. *Journal of Surgical Education.* 2008;65(2):157.

163. Magnetic Resonance Technology Information Portal. Superparamagnetic Iron Oxide. http://www.mr-tip.com/serv1. php?type=db1&dbs=Superparamagnetic%20Iron%20Oxide. Accessed March 24, 2011.

164. Freitas RA Jr. What is Nanomedicine? *Nanomedicine: Nanotechnology, Biology, and Medicine.* 2005;1(1):5.

165. Sershen SR, Westcott SL, Halas NJ, West JL. Temperature-sensitive polymer-nanoshell composite for photothermally modulated drug delivery. *Journal of Biomedical Materials Research.* 2000;51(3):293–298.

166. Kimball JW. Kimball's Biology Page. Kimball's Biology Page website. http://users.rcn.com/jkimball.ma.ultranet/ BiologyPages/. Accessed April 1, 2011.

167. Ruoff RS, Kadish KM, eds. Fullerenes: recent advances in the chemistry and physics of fullerenes and related materials. Pennington, NJ: Electrochemical Society Press; 1997:989–990.

168. Leoni L, Desai TA. Nonporous biocapsules for the encapsulation of insulinoma cells: biotransport and biocompatibility considerations. *IEEE Trans Biomed Engineering.* 2001;48(11):1335–1341.

169. Freitas RA Jr. What is Nanomedicine? *Nanomedicine: Nanotechnology, Biology, and Medicine.* 2005;1(1):331.

170. Freitas, RA Jr. What is Nanomedicine? *Nanotechnology, Biology, and Medicine.* 2005;1(1):2–9.

171. Staggers N, McCasky T, Brazelton N, Kennedy R. Nanotechnology: the coming revolution and its implications for consumers, clinicians, and informatics. *Nursing Outlook.* 2008;56(5):268.

172. The National Nanotechnology Initiative. Research and development leading to a revolution in technology and Industry: Supplement to the President's FY 2008 Budget. Washington, DC: The US Government; 2007:6.

173. Freitas RA Jr. What is Nanomedicine? *Nanomedicine: Nanotechnology, Biology, and Medicine.* 2005;(1):325.

Index